# BMA

# Expecting Trouble

## Early Warnings and Rapid Responses in Maternal Medical Care

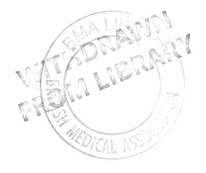

# Expecting Trouble

## Early Warnings and Rapid Responses in Maternal Medical Care

Edited by
Lauren A. Plante, MD, MPH

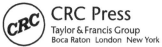

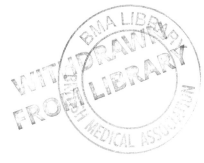

CRC Press
Taylor & Francis Group
Boca Raton  London  New York

CRC Press is an imprint of the
Taylor & Francis Group, an **informa** business

CRC Press
Taylor & Francis Group
6000 Broken Sound Parkway NW, Suite 300
Boca Raton, FL 33487-2742

© 2018 by Taylor & Francis Group, LLC
CRC Press is an imprint of Taylor & Francis Group, an Informa business

No claim to original U.S. Government works

Printed on acid-free paper by Ashford Colour Press Ltd.

International Standard Book Number-13: 978-1-4987-4768-4 (Paperback)
International Standard Book Number-13: 978-0-8153-7973-7 (Hardback)

---

**Library of Congress Cataloging-in-Publication Data**

---

Names: Plante, Lauren A., editor.
Title: Expecting trouble : early warnings and rapid responses in maternal
medical care / edited by Lauren A. Plante.
Other titles: Expecting trouble (Plante) | Early warnings and rapid responses
in maternal medical care
Description: Boca Raton, FL : CRC Press/Taylor & Francis Group, [2018] |
Includes bibliographical references and index.
Identifiers: LCCN 2017039172| ISBN 9780815379737 (hardback : alk. paper) |
ISBN 9781498747684 (pbk. : alk. paper) | ISBN 9781351215145 (ebook)
Subjects: | MESH: Pregnancy Complications--therapy | Critical Care--methods |
Early Diagnosis | Hospital Rapid Response Team
Classification: LCC RG571 | NLM WQ 240 | DDC 618.2/025--dc23
LC record available at https://lccn.loc.gov/2017039172

---

**Visit the Taylor & Francis Web site at**
**http://www.taylorandfrancis.com**

**and the CRC Press Web site at**
**http://www.crcpress.com**

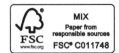

*This book is dedicated to my mother, Jean, who survived severe postpartum hemorrhage;*

*to my daughter, Aislinn, who I hope will never have need of any of the interventions here;*

*and to my son, Kieran, with the wish that nothing herein ever hits close to home.*

# Contents

# *Preface*

The genesis of this book derives from an intern's first weekend on call, when she found herself inadequate to the task of pronouncing a patient dead, having failed to prevent that outcome.

Most in-hospital mortality is preceded by one or more signals, which, if identified and corrected, would have the potential to prevent that outcome. This is the premise that underlies early warning systems. In obstetrical care, too, maternal early warning systems have been developed. A systematic pattern of observations is implemented, at a preset schedule. If an abnormal signal is detected, a response is required. The patient is evaluated and steps are taken to correct the condition. So early warning systems must be coupled with strategies for rapid responses. Many institutions have developed rapid response teams for specific situations (e.g., cardiac arrest, major obstetric hemorrhage), but this is not true everywhere, nor does it relieve the first responder of the responsibility once the team has been called.

The goal of this book is to provide you with responses to some of these warning signals. While it is true that not all signs or symptoms inevitably predict deterioration, all the signals discussed in this book should trigger an evaluation at the bedside; the only way to distinguish alarm from false alarm is to further investigate. Is more than one response possible? Of course, but having a list of precompiled responses is useful in emergencies. Depending on your practice setting, you may not see any of these so often that you have already developed your own responses.

The book is organized in such a way that it can be useful as a quick reference. After introductory chapters on both early warning systems and rapid response teams, the rest of the book is devoted to signs or symptoms that should be taken seriously. If you are called to see a pregnant or postpartum patient because she is hypertensive, complaining of dyspnea, or potentially in some other kind of trouble, you should have both a differential diagnosis and a rapid response available to the presenting condition. In the most acute situations, it will often be necessary to simultaneously treat and work up, while in other cases, there may be time to work through the diagnosis more deliberatively.

Having evaluated the patient, if the most severe, life-threatening conditions are ruled out, there is time for an extensive differential diagnosis, although that is, unfortunately, somewhat beyond the scope of this endeavor. It may also turn out that the presenting complaint is an exaggeration of normal symptoms of pregnancy; for example, subjective complaints of dyspnea are common in pregnancy and are not always indicative of pathology. But it is important to exclude the more dangerous possibilities rather than to simply assume that they are not in play.

Most pregnancy is medically uneventful. Nevertheless, maternal mortality has been increasing in the United States, alone among high-income nations. Multiple explanations have been advanced, from changes in demographics (age, obesity, medical comorbidities), to rising cesarean rates, to inequities in access to care. These explanations will not help you at the bedside. But, on the individual level, being prepared for the possibility of acute decompensation has the potential to save women's lives. Expect trouble and know how to respond when you identify it.

# Contributors

**Sandra Asanjarani, RNC, MS, NP**
Perinatal Safety Specialist
Department of Maternal Child Health Nursing
New York Presbyterian Queens
Flushing, New York

**K. Ashley Brandt, DO**
Associate Clinical Faculty
Department of Obstetrics and Gynecology
Drexel University College of Medicine
Philadelphia, Pennsylvania
and
Department of Obstetrics and Gynecology
Phoenixville Hospital
Phoenixville, Pennsylvania

**Casey Brown, DO**
Department of Obstetrics and Gynecology
Lehigh Valley Health Network
Allentown, Pennsylvania

**Hugh M. Ehrenberg, MD**
College of Medicine
Drexel University
Philadelphia, Pennsylvania
and
Maternal Fetal Medicine
Crozer-Keystone Health Network
Crozer Chester Medical Center
Upland, Pennsylvania

**Nadir El-Sharawi, MBBS**
Department of Anesthesiology
University of Arkansas for Medical Sciences
Little Rock, Arkansas

**Amanda Flicker, MD**
Department of Obstetrics and Gynecology
Lehigh Valley Health Network
Allentown, Pennsylvania
and
Department of Obstetrics and Gynecology
University of South Florida
Morsani College of Medicine
Tampa, Florida

**Victoria Greenberg, MD**
Department of Obstetrics and Gynecology and
    Center for Women and Children's Health
    Research
Christiana Care Health System
Newark, Delaware

**Nicole Ruddock Hall, MD**
Georgia Perinatal Consultants
Atlanta, Georgia

**Afshan B. Hameed, MD, FACC, FACOG**
Division of Maternal Fetal Medicine
Department of Obstetrics and Gynecology
and
Division of Cardiology
Department of Medicine
University of California
Irvine, California

**Matthew K. Hoffman, MD, MPH, FACOG**
Marie E. Pinizzotto, MD
Department of Obstetrics and Gynecology and
    Center for Women and Children's Health
    Research
Christiana Care Health System
Newark, Delaware

**Jhenette Lauder, MD**
Department of Obstetrics and Gynecology
Christiana Hospital
Newark, Delaware

**Lawrence Leeman, MD, MPH**
Department of Family and Community Medicine
    and Department of Obstetrics and Gynecology
University of New Mexico
Albuquerque, New Mexico

**Stephanie Martin, DO**
Medical Director
Clinical Concepts in Obstetrics
Scottsdale, Arizona

**Brigid McCue, MD, PhD**
Ob/Gyn Hospitalist Division
Ochsner Health System
New Orleans, Louisiana

**Jill M. Mhyre, MD**
Department of Anesthesiology
University of Arkansas for Medical Sciences
Little Rock, Arkansas

**Gayle Olson Koutrouvelis, MD**
Division of Maternal Fetal Medicine
Department of Obstetrics and Gynecology
University of Texas Medical Branch
Galveston, Texas

**Lauren A. Plante, MD, MPH**
Division of Maternal Fetal Medicine
Department of Obstetrics and Gynecology
    and Department of Anesthesiology
College of Medicine
Drexel University
Philadelphia, Pennsylvania

**Anna Maya Powell, MD**
Clinical Instructor, Obstetrics and Gynecology
Medical University of South Carolina
Charleston, South Carolina

**Anthony Sciscione, DO**
Department of Obstetrics and Gynecology
Christiana Hospital
Newark, Delaware

**Neil S. Seligman, MD**
Division of Maternal Fetal Medicine
Department of Obstetrics & Gynecology
University of Rochester Medical Center
Rochester, New York

**Daniel W. Skupski, MD**
Professor of Obstetrics & Gynecology
Weill Cornell Medicine
Chairman, Obstetrics and Gynecology
Director, Maternal Fetal Medicine
New York Presbyterian Queens
Flushing, New York

**John C. Smulian, MD, MPH**
Department of Obstetrics and Gynecology
Lehigh Valley Health Network
Allentown, Pennsylvania
and
Department of Obstetrics and Gynecology
University of South Florida
Morsani College of Medicine
Tampa, Florida

**Arthur Jason Vaught, MD**
Assistant Professor
Department of Gynecology and Obstetrics
and
Maternal Fetal Medicine
Department of Surgery
Surgical Critical Care
Baltimore, Maryland

**Melissa Westermann, MD**
Division of Maternal Fetal Medicine
Department of Obstetrics and Gynecology
University of California
Irvine, California

**Nicole Yonke, MD, MPH**
Department of Family and Community Medicine
University of New Mexico
Albuquerque, New Mexico

# 1

# *Maternal Early Warning Systems in Obstetrics*

**Nadir El-Sharawi, MBBS and Jill M. Mhyre, MD**

## CONTENTS

## Introduction

Critical illness is relatively rare in pregnant and postpartum women, but can rapidly evolve. Early detection allows for timely and potentially life-saving treatment. Unfortunately, delays in recognition and diagnosis are frequently identified in maternal mortality reviews. The 2003–2005 Report on Confidential Enquiries into Maternal Deaths in the United Kingdom (1) highlighted cases where the early warning signs of maternal collapse went unrecognized. The California Pregnancy-Associated Mortality Review Committee (2) suggested that 41% of maternal deaths had a good to strong chance of being prevented with improvements in clinical care. Across a range of lethal diagnoses that included preeclampsia, hemorrhage, sepsis, and heart failure, delayed response to abnormal vital sign triggers was the most common missed opportunity to avoid the fatal outcome (2).

Early signs of acute physiological deterioration in pregnant and peripartum women are difficult to recognize. Pregnancy is characterized by marked changes in the cardiovascular and respiratory systems, so new symptoms such as shortness of breath and fatigue can be dismissed as normal. Most pregnant women have uneventful pregnancies, and serious complications are relatively rare. Healthy pregnant women frequently mount a robust response to underlying illness. Particularly with sepsis and hemorrhage, maternal blood pressure and mentation can be preserved at the expense of surging catecholamine levels.

Early detection followed by a timely and competent clinical response in women with serious illness is crucial in improving clinical outcomes. The Joint Commission (3) published a *Sentential Event Alert* on maternal death in the United States in 2010. It required that hospitals "develop written criteria describing early warning signs of a change or deterioration in a patient's condition and when to seek further assistance" and "have a process for recognizing and responding as soon as a patient's condition appears to be worsening" (3).

## What Is an Early Warning System?

An early warning system (EWS) is a protocol designed to identify patients who are at risk of complications or impending medical deterioration and to secure skilled clinical help by the bedside. The original EWS measured patient physiological variables such as pulse rate, respiratory rate, systolic blood pressure, and level of consciousness. A predetermined value was assigned to each physiological variable dependent upon the extent of deviation from the normal (4). Physiological observations are regularly monitored; if one variable reaches a defined threshold, then an automatic response is initiated to expedite early assessment and intervention by a suitable qualified clinician.

EWSs can be categorized into the following:

1. Simple triggering systems – Where one positive parameter triggers the response.
2. Scoring systems – Where multiple physiological parameters are given a cumulative score. The value of the score triggers the response and determines the level of escalation that is required.

The advantage of the simple trigger system is its simplicity. Only one abnormal parameter is required to activate the call for help. The simple scoring system is more reliable, less prone to calculation errors, and has improved reproducibility (5,6). Such practical factors may be important in allowing widespread implementation in various hospital and community settings. The main disadvantage of such a system is that it does not easily lend itself to risk stratification or allow a graded response that occurs with scoring systems. There is also some suggestion that an aggregate weighted scoring system may be more sensitive in detecting early decompensation, because multiple minor abnormalities may occur before a single physiological parameter is sufficiently abnormal to trigger a clinician evaluation (7). Furthermore, this type of scoring system requires the full set of vital sign parameters to be documented in order to calculate the total score. By collecting the entire set of physiological variables in this way, it is less likely that any single measurement will be missed.

## Nonobstetric Early Warning Systems

Many early warning scoring systems are available. They have been used in numerous specialities in various forms including general surgery, medicine, and pediatrics (8–10). However, there remains a lack of standardization and consistency. Numerous scoring systems lack appropriate methodology, statistical power, and evidence regarding their benefit (11). The different EWSs are therefore not necessarily equivalent or interchangeable. "Put simply, when assessing acutely ill patients using these various scores, we are not speaking the same language and this can lead to a lack of consistency in the approach to detection and response to acute illness" (12). To deal with some of these concerns, the Royal College of Physicians in the United Kingdom devised the National Early Warning Score (NEWS). The NEWS has been adopted as the national standard for nonpregnant adults and has been evaluated against a variety of other EWSs. NEWS was found to be more sensitive than most existing systems and just as good at discriminating the risk of acute mortality or better. Nonobstetric EWSs are not appropriate for the obstetric setting, because they do not account for the physiological changes of pregnancy. As an example, in the NEWS, the normal range for systolic blood pressure is 111–219 mmHg. For pregnant women with preeclampsia, systolic blood pressure measurements above 160 mmHg are abnormal and should be treated to reduce the risk of hemorrhagic stroke. Values as low as 90 mmHg are frequently normal.

## Maternal Early Warning Systems

Maternal EWSs are modified to account for the normal physiological changes of pregnancy and to specifically detect the unique disease processes in the pregnant parturient. There are five main pathological conditions that cause the vast majority of severe maternal morbidity and mortality in pregnancy and the postpartum period. These include the following:

- Hemorrhage
- Sepsis
- Hypertensive disorders

- Cardiovascular dysfunction
- Venous thromboembolism

All scoring systems must balance sensitivity and specificity to most accurately identify those patients who are most likely to benefit from increased medical attention. For maternal EWSs, sensitivity is the percentage of women who trigger the scoring tool out of the total population of women who have physiological deterioration. When a tool has high sensitivity, it is reasonable to rule out pathology among those women who do not trigger the scoring tool. Specificity is the percentage of women who do not trigger the scoring tool, out of women who are perfectly well. Positive predictive value is the number of true alerts, meaning the percentage of women who are becoming sick out of all those who trigger the scoring tool. Because maternal deterioration is rare, specificity must be extremely high in order to maintain a reasonable positive predictive value and avoid a large number of false positive alerts. If the majority of alerts are false positives, this can overburden the clinical team, and lead to "alarm fatigue" and a tendency to dismiss subsequent triggering events. Thus, specificity is particularly important to ensure a high-functioning maternal EWS.

In addition, the ideal EWS would possess the following characteristics:

- Ease of use
- Widespread compliance among nursing, midwifery, and medical staff
- The ability to identify relevant clinical indicators of patient deterioration
- Trigger a timely and competent response plan when activated
- Supported by evidence of a reduction in patient morbidity and mortality

Numerous maternal EWSs have been proposed; however, there remains no widespread agreement on what criteria should be included and what level of abnormality should trigger a clinician response or what that response should be (13).

The 2007 Confidential Enquiry report (1) recommended the use of the modified early obstetric warning system (MEOWS) to help in the more timely recognition, treatment, and referral of women who have or are developing a critical illness. Shown in Table 1.1 is the MEOWS, a simple scoring system which defines various physiological parameters that should be measured at regular intervals; a clinical response is triggered when two moderately abnormal parameters (yellow alerts) or one extremely abnormal parameter (red alert) is triggered. Singh et al. (14) conducted a validation study to assess MEOWS triggers as a predictor for morbidity. Six hundred seventy-six patients were evaluated using MEOWS. Thirteen percent of patients suffered morbidity and 30% had a positive MEOWS trigger. The study revealed a MEOWS sensitivity of 89% for predicting morbidity, a specificity of 79%, and a positive predictive value of 39%. Consequently, 6 of every 10 triggering events was for a woman experiencing normal birth.

TABLE 1.1

Modified Early Obstetric Warning System

| Physiological Parameter | Yellow Alert | Red Alert |
|---|---|---|
| Respiration rate | 21–30 | <10 or >30 |
| Oxygen saturation | | <95 |
| Temperature | 35–36 | <35 or >38 |
| Systolic blood pressure | 150–160 or 90–100 | <90 or >160 |
| Diastolic blood pressure | 90–100 | >100 |
| Heart rate | 100–120 or 40–50 | >120 or <40 |
| Pain score | 2–3 | |
| Neurological response | Voice | Unresponsive, pain |

TABLE 1.2

Maternal Early Warning Criteria, Triggers

| Physiological Parameter | Trigger |
|---|---|
| Respiration rate (breaths per min) | <10 or >30 |
| Oxygen saturation on room air at sea level (%) | <95 |
| Systolic blood pressure (mmHg) | <90 or >160 |
| Diastolic blood pressure (mmHg) | >110 |
| Heart rate (beats per min) | <50 or >120 |
| Oliguria (mL/hour) ≥2 hours | <30 |
| Maternal agitation, confusion, or unresponsiveness; patient with hypertension reporting a nonremitting headache or shortness of breath | |

Carle et al. (15) used a national database of intensive care unit (ICU) admissions in the United Kingdom to empirically derive a maternal early warning score. For each physiological parameter studied, the authors recorded the most abnormal value measured during the first 24 hours of ICU admission. Multivariable modeling identified the panel of parameters that most accurately predicted subsequent death. The empirically devised mathematical model demonstrated excellent accuracy to predict patient deterioration and mortality in a second group of women, but did not perform better than the more clinically meaningful MEOWS parameters that were recommended by the Confidential Enquiry report published in 2007 (1). The EWS published by Carle et al. has not been validated within the maternity ward. The authors concluded that a simplified scoring system had similar accuracy and was more likely to be suited to a labor ward environment.

Currently, the Oxford Biomedical Research Centre (16) in the United Kingdom is recruiting participants in the Oxford 4P study (pregnancy, physiology, pattern prediction) to capture the normal distributions of physiological data in "low-risk" pregnancies from 14 weeks' gestation to 2 weeks postpartum in order to develop an evidence-based EWS. Measurements greater than two standard deviations from the mean will be defined as abnormal for the purpose of directing medical attention.

In 2014, a multidisciplinary working group, the National Partnership for Maternal Safety developed the Maternal Early Warning Criteria (MEWC), shown in Table 1.2 (17). This simple trigger system was based on the MEOWS "red alert" physiological parameters; any single abnormal parameter will initiate a bedside evaluation from a qualified clinician. The MEWC reflects observations among maternal death reviews in the United States that prolonged episodes of frankly abnormal vital signs precede a number of maternal deaths. By focusing on red alert values, the MEWC is designed to maximize specificity, to avoid high rates of false positive alerts, and to support a culture in which abnormal vital signs are taken seriously. The single parameter system was chosen to facilitate rapid and widespread implementation within the whole spectrum of delivery centers from small community hospitals to large academic institutions.

A recent study aimed at determining whether predefined physiological parameters (referred to as maternal early warning triggers) can predict maternal morbidity. The presence of two or more maternal early warning triggers lasting 30 minutes or more had a specificity of 96% for predicting patient morbidity (18). Therefore, multiple and progressively abnormal vital signs are more accurate than single measurements for identifying patients with impending critical illness. Clinical staff should be trained to recognize and respond to trends that represent significant deterioration.

## Clinical Response to Maternal Early Warning Systems

Of the EWSs described earlier, the MEOWS has become the national standard in the United Kingdom as recommended by the Centre for Maternal and Child Enquiries. In the United States, the National Council for Patient Safety has suggested the use of the MEWC. Whichever surveillance is used, an effective escalation policy is required.

Mhyre et al. (17) propose the following when an EWS is triggered:

1. Prompt reporting to a physician or other qualified clinician
2. Prompt bedside evaluation by a physician or other qualified clinician with the ability to activate resources in order to initiate emergency diagnostic and therapeutic interventions as needed

Due to the variety of different clinical care settings, local policy specific to the needs of each obstetric unit would dictate the desired escalation plan. Regardless, multidisciplinary communication is essential, and the specific protocol for system activation needs to be well defined in advance, including the following:

1. How to trigger the alarm (e.g., abbreviated communication, mobile communication, automated paging device)
2. Who to notify and who will respond (e.g., obstetric provider, anesthesiologist, medical emergency team)
3. How quickly to expect a response
4. When and how to activate the clinical chain of command in order to ensure an appropriate response
5. The frequency of further clinical monitoring and subsequent resuscitative measures while awaiting a response
6. The components of an effective response; as a minimum, this should be a bedside evaluation as opposed to phone-based management

To actually improve clinical outcomes, a trigger must lead to prompt bedside evaluation and a clinical treatment pathway. These treatment pathways should focus on early recognition and treatment of the underlying pathology with an emphasis on a team response.

As an example, the Maternal Early Warning Trigger (MEWT) tool links abnormal vital sign parameters with specific care pathways and recommendations for patient assessment and treatment. The MEWT tool was designed to specifically screen for sepsis, hemorrhage, preeclampsia, and cardiovascular dysfunction, which are the major causes of maternal morbidity. The clinical responses are separated into treatment pathways or care bundles depending on which physiological parameters are triggered. Emerging evidence suggests that the MEWT system does reduce maternal morbidity (19).

Activation protocols can be tested using team simulations and training. This has the added advantage of identifying and solving any underlying system problems.

## Implementation of Early Warning Systems

Maternal EWSs provide a structure to identify and evaluate early patient deterioration, but effective implementation requires a high-functioning team with a commitment to a culture of safety. For successful implementation, all medical and nursing personnel need to understand their role and the importance of following the protocol as a team. The implementation process should begin when clinical and managerial leaderships are ready and have bought in to the concept.

Physicians and nurses interpret data from EWSs differently depending upon their clinical background and priorities (20). It is essential that leaders from the multidisciplinary team communicate their commitment, as there are numerous cultural and institutional factors to overcome. Nursing staff may deem the recording of MEWS parameters as inconvenient and unnecessary especially if there is already widespread duplication within the medical notes. It is not uncommon for the perceived value of an MEWS system to be questioned in the light of increased workload commitments, low prevalence of complications, and excessive medical intervention. Tools embedded within the electronic medical records can minimize the disruption to nursing workflow, reduce calculation errors and provide a process for easier implementation. This can be taken one step further with full automation of MEWS, which would allow triggers to be adjusted according to different hospital settings and automatic notification of the response team. Nevertheless, unfiltered automated triggering systems can result in an extremely high rate of false positive alerts, all of which require clinical interpretation.

False alarms can be a nuisance to the team members and can easily prompt haphazard and ineffective implementation. Nurses chastised for bothering senior clinicians will delay notification in subsequent cases (21). Strong leadership among service leaders, hospital administrators, and senior clinicians should promote prompt notification and timely bedside assessment as the norm, whatever the clinical outcome, without fear of reprimand. To minimize the rate of false positive alerts, a warning system with high specificity should be chosen and should incorporate the subjective judgments of health professionals. Abnormal parameters may reflect measurement artifact, so nurses should be trained to verify the measurement with a senior nurse. Progressively abnormal values, those that persist for at least 30 minutes, and multiple abnormal physiological parameters are more likely to represent true clinical deterioration. A standardized training program would allow healthcare staff to understand the significance of the system and the local policies in place for responding to the trigger.

Insufficient staffing levels and increasing workload may lead to the misuse of MEWS, especially when the obstetric census is high. In academic facilities, junior doctors are often the first to be notified when a MEWS is triggered. Most junior doctors have an overwhelming workload, and MEWS can be misused as a severity score to prioritize their work (20). As such, it is important to identify a series of qualified clinicians who could respond to a request for a timely bedside review, backed up by a team-based response for patients with rapid clinical decline, e.g., obstetric emergency response team.

If the bedside assessment by the evaluating clinician indicates normal physiology for the patient or the diagnosis remains unclear, then a customized plan regarding the frequency of observation and further assessment needs to be established with the bedside nurse. This may involve altering the parameter trigger if all diagnostic investigations are normal and acute illness has been ruled out. The MEWS should be used for the initial assessment of acute illness and continuously monitored throughout the entire inpatient stay.

When optimally implemented, MEWS identify those women who are most likely to benefit from medical attention. But to improve maternal safety, every MEWS relies on astute clinicians to make accurate and timely diagnoses and to treat the underlying cause of the illness. To that end, the culture of clinical evaluation should change from one in which clinicians wait for illness to become evident, to one in which EWS triggers prompt the evaluating clinician to consider a relevant differential diagnosis, and to rule out the most likely life-threatening diagnoses. For example, if a patient demonstrates sustained tachycardia (over 120 beats per minute) following cesarean delivery, then concealed hemorrhage must be excluded, and orthostatic hypotension, uterine tone, lochia, abdominal ultrasound, and hemoglobin levels should be evaluated. But if all values are normal and tachycardia persists, then less common diagnoses should be considered (e.g., heart failure, sepsis, venous thromboembolism).

Diagnosis can be difficult. Sometimes, the trigger is little more than a sense by the patient, the family, or her nurse that "something is wrong." Subtle maternal confusion can persist for days before pneumonia becomes evident, and in that time, it can become easy to dismiss the patient as simply confused. The point of the MEWS is to strategically evaluate and to continue to observe the patient with abnormal triggers, even when no diagnosis is established, especially when no diagnosis has been established. This book is written for all clinicians called upon to respond to an EWS trigger. Each chapter details an evaluation strategy for specific abnormal clinical findings. Taken together, high-functioning maternal EWSs, smart clinicians, and the contents of this book have the potential to improve the safety of our maternal health systems and to profoundly improve the lives of the families we serve.

## REFERENCES

1. Lewis, G (ed) 2007. The Confidential Enquiry into Maternal and Child Health (CEMCH). Saving Mothers' Lives: Reviewing maternal deaths to make motherhood safer – 2003-2005. The Seventh Report on Confidential Enquiries into Maternal Deaths in the United Kingdom. London: CEMACH.
2. Main EK, McCain CL, Morton CH, Holtby S, Lawton ES. Pregnancy-related mortality in California: Causes, characteristics, and improvement opportunities. *Obstet Gynecol.* 2015; 125(4):938-947.

3. Joint Commission on Accreditation of Healthcare Organizations (JCAHO), USA. Preventing maternal death. *Sentin Event Alert.* 2010; 44:1-4.

4. Goldhill DR, McNarry AF, Mandersloot G, McGinley A. A physiologically-based early warning score for ward patients: The association between score and outcome. *Anaesthesia.* 2005; 60(6):547-553.

5. Goldhill DR, Worthington L, Mulcahy A, Tarling M, Sumner A. The patient-at-risk team: Identifying and managing seriously ill ward patients. *Anaesthesia.* 1999; 54(9):853-860.

6. Subbe CP, Gao H, Harrison DA. Reproducibility of physiological track-and-trigger warning systems for identifying at-risk patients on the ward. *Intensive Care Med.* 2007; 33(4):619-624.

7. Hands C, Reid E, Meredith P, Smith GB, Prytherch DR, Schmidt PE et al. Patterns in the recording of vital signs and early warning scores: Compliance with a clinical escalation protocol. *BMJ Qual Safety.* 2013; 22(9):719-726.

8. Seiger N, Maconochie I, Oostenbrink R, Moll HA. Validity of different pediatric early warning scores in the emergency department. *Pediatrics.* 2013; 132(4):e841-e850.

9. Smith ME, Chiovaro JC, O'Neil M, Kansagara D, Quinones AR, Freeman M et al. Early warning system scores for clinical deterioration in hospitalized patients: A systematic review. *Ann Amer Thorac Soc.* 2014; 11(9):1454-1465.

10. Patel MS, Jones MA, Jiggins M, Williams SC. Does the use of a "track and trigger" warning system reduce mortality in trauma patients? *Injury.* 2011; 42(12):1455-1459.

11. McGaughey J, Alderdice F, Fowler R, Kapila A, Mayhew A, Moutray M. Outreach and Early Warning Systems (EWS) for the prevention of intensive care admission and death of critically ill adult patients on general hospital wards. *Cochrane Database Syst Rev.* 2007; Jul 18 (3):Cd005529.

12. Williams B, Alberti G, Ball C, Bell D, Binks R, Durham L. *National Early Warning Score (NEWS): Standardising the assessment of acute-illness severity in the NHS.* London: The Royal College of Physicians; 2012.

13. Friedman AM. Maternal early warning systems. *Obstet Gynecol Clin North Am.* 2015; 42(2):289-298.

14. Singh S, McGlennan A, England A, Simons R. A validation study of the CEMACH recommended modified early obstetric warning system (MEOWS). *Anaesthesia.* 2012; 67(1):12-18.

15. Carle C, Alexander P, Columb M, Johal J. Design and internal validation of an obstetric early warning score: Secondary analysis of the Intensive Care National Audit and Research Centre Case Mix Programme database. *Anaesthesia.* 2013; 68(4):354-367.

16. Kumar F, Kemp J, Edwards C, Pullon RM, Loerup L, Triantafyllidis A, Salvi D, Gibson O, Gerry S, MacKillop LH, Tarassenko L, Watkinson, PJ. Pregnancy physiology pattern prediction study (4P study): Protocol of an observational cohort study collecting vital sign information to inform the development of an accurate centile-based obstetric early warning score. *BMJ Open.* 2017 Sep 1;7(9):e016034.

17. Mhyre JM, D'Oria R, Hameed AB, Lappen JR, Holley SL, Hunter SK et al. The maternal early warning criteria: A proposal from the national partnership for maternal safety. *J Obstet Gynecol Neonatal Nurs.* 2014; 43(6):771-779.

18. Hedriana HL, Wiesner S, Downs BG, Pelletreau B, Shields LE. Baseline assessment of a hospital-specific early warning trigger system for reducing maternal morbidity. *I J Gynecol Obstet.* 2016; 132(3): 337-341.

19. Shields LE, Wiesner S, Klein C, Pelletreau B, Hedriana HL. Use of Maternal Early Warning Trigger tool reduces maternal morbidity. *Am J Obstet Gynecol.* 2016; 214(4):527.e1-6.

20. Greaves J, Greaves D, Gallagher H, Steven A, Pearson P. Doctors and nurses have different priorities in using the Modified Early Warning Score protocol. *Br J Anaesth.* 2016; 116(2):298.

21. Considine J, Botti M. Who, when and where? Identification of patients at risk of an in-hospital adverse event: Implications for nursing practice. *In J Nurs Pract.* 2004; 10(1):21-31.

# 2

# Rapid Response Teams

**Gayle Olson Koutrouvelis, MD**

The concept of improving patient outcomes through the use of early warning systems most likely originated in 1999, when Goldhill et al. (1) identified physiological parameters that manifested in patients prior to the need for admission to intensive care units (ICUs). This concept gained support when others also noted that the early identification and correction of abnormal physiology may not only improve outcome but may also avoid morbidity altogether (2).

Rapid response teams (RRTs) were highlighted in 2004 when the Institute of Health Care Improvement championed the "Save 100,000 Lives" campaign and listed RRTs as one of the six initiatives for improving quality of patient care (3). The American College of Obstetricians and Gynecologists (4) also promoted RRTs as a key strategy to improve outcomes. RRTs are a component of rapid response systems (RRSs); the RRT includes a group of individuals who provide a rapid response to patients who demonstrate predetermined signs and symptoms from a predetermined set of clinical criteria, suggestive of clinical deterioration. The RRS includes the RRT plus the whole-hospital approach to improving, recognizing, and managing patients who are at risk for clinical deterioration (5). The initial culture of RRS and RRT desired to reduce adverse events primarily surrounding cardiac arrests, unplanned admissions to ICUs, and unexpected deaths of inpatients. Decreases in all-cause mortality have been more difficult to demonstrate because the patients most likely to cause the activation of RRTs are likely to be the most ill. Nonetheless, an overall reduction in mortality by as much as 23% has been documented in some reviews of RRTs (5). Additional benefits of RRT and RRS include clarifications of care, expert opinions on end-of-life care, facilitation of ICU transfers, and development of continuous monitoring systems (5).

A core goal for an intervention by an RRT is that the program promptly brings individuals with critical care or advanced skills to the bedside (6). In order to be effective, the RRT should be activated shortly after a trigger is identified, and longer lag times are associated with higher mortality (7). This means RRT providers should be immediately available on site. The RRT does not replace the primary care physician, but functions during an acute event and returns the patient to the primary care team once the patient is stabilized (6).

The composition of the RRT can vary depending on the population demographic and ethnic distribution, hospital location, level of acuity, and available resources (8). For some hospitals, a physician member could be represented by a hospitalist, critical care physician, or nonphysician extenders (nurse practitioner, physician assistant).

In nonobstetric adult populations, parameters that might activate an RRT response include acute respiratory or cardiac failure, severe hypertension or hypotension, pulmonary edema, and sepsis (8), while in an obstetric population, an RRT could respond to similar parameters plus obstetrics-specific situations such as fetal bradycardia, postpartum hemorrhage, and shoulder dystocia (4). Thus, the concept that RRTs intervene for early warning signs that precede adverse health outcomes has been extended to the obstetric population. In 2007, Lewis (9) led a confidential obstetric audit of maternal deaths reported in the United Kingdom and used what was learned from maternal tragedies to set practice recommendations. The use of a modified early obstetric warning system (MEOWS) was one of these recommendations (9,10).

In 2012, a prospective observational study of MEOWS enrolled 673 inpatient women between 20 weeks gestation to 6 weeks postpartum, using physiological parameters of temperature, systolic blood pressure, diastolic blood pressure, heart rate, respiratory rate, oxygen saturation, pain score, and mental status. Thirty percent of the subjects had parameters that activated a trigger, and 3% fitted the criteria for morbidity, the most common parameters being hemorrhage, hypertension, and infection. There were no intensive care admissions, cardiac arrests, or deaths. The overall sensitivity for MEOWS in predicting morbidity was 89% (95% confidence interval [CI]: 81–95%); specificity, 79% (95% CI: 76–82%); positive predictive value, 39% (95% CI: 32–46%); and negative predictive value, 98% (95% CI: 96–99%) (11). In a second prospective observational study including 1065 women between the 28th week of pregnancy and 6 weeks postpartum, similar physiological parameters were identified as triggers but were blinded to the caregivers, and patients were only managed according to routine hospital protocols. Subjects with physiological parameters that fell into trigger zones were more likely to experience instrumental delivery, cesarean section, blood transfusions, and adverse composite neonatal outcomes. In this second study, the MEOWS chart was found to be 86.4% sensitive and 85.2% specific and have positive and negative predictive values of 54 and 97%, respectively, for predicting obstetric morbidity (10). Both studies support the use of parameters and triggers to identify early stages of acute compromise, allowing for potential intervention and change in outcome. Both demonstrate benefit from an early warning system in obstetrics. The Royal College of Anaesthetists has proposed a uniform national early warning score for obstetric patients in the UK, analogous to the National Early Warning Score used there for nonpregnant adults in the acute hospital setting, with physiological triggers adapted for pregnancy norms (12).

Establishing an RRT is a multistep process and involves multidisciplinary members. All components of the process must be considered, including clinicians, nurses, support staff, page operators, blood bank, and other ancillary services. The outcome of interest, early warning parameters, and trigger values are identified. RRT member roles, debriefings, training, feedback, administrative oversight, and governance are all needed for a sustainable RRT (4). The components of the RRT can be organized into an afferent limb, primarily consisting of activators; triggers; and adjuncts, enabling successful activation, and an efferent limb which includes responders. Both limbs communicate and interrelate to administration, quality improvement, and governance (4,7). In general, activators, as the term suggests, activate or pull the trigger, setting the efferent arm in motion, which is the response team attending to the patient. Activators and responders may vary depending on the facility. For example, patients, family members, nurses, and aides may serve as activators, while house staff, hospitalists, critical care physicians, nurses, nurse practitioners, and respiratory therapists may be included as responders. It is important for each institution to design the RRT that works best for them. In addition, communication skills, debriefing, feedback from responders, and continuing training should be routine components of each RRT, particularly after an activation has taken place (4). A conceptual diagram for an RRT is presented in Figure 2.1. Obstetric patients present a unique challenge for RRTs because they are usually younger and healthier and do not manifest the same set of critical events as do nonobstetric critically ill adult patients. However, life-threatening situations can develop, often with much less warning than is available for the nonpregnant adult. This can be a barrier to a successful sustainable obstetric RRT. Key components for successful and sustainable obstetric RRTs have been designed and described by Richardson et al. (13). This obstetric emergency team (OBET) is similar in design to what has been described in other settings and includes afferent and efferent limbs, effective communication, multidisciplinary members, feedback, and support from interprofessional leadership (13). In this report, indications for the activation of the OBET included triggers related to external fetal monitoring abnormalities (58%), precipitous delivery (14.3%), and postpartum hemorrhage (8.7%) (13). Finally, a "response dose" has been considered for use as a standard utilization metric for RRTs. The response dose is described as the number of RRS activation calls per 1000 admissions. The response dose should match or exceed the frequency of the problem, and if the dose is insufficient, there will be little effect on adverse outcomes. At this time, an optimal response dose for an obstetric emergency team could not be determined.

RRTs, along with the broader scope of a hospital culture of rapid response systems, have the potential to improve patient care and decrease mortality. In addition, there may be a reduction in triage errors and an increase in patient flow management, all which serve to improve outcomes (13).

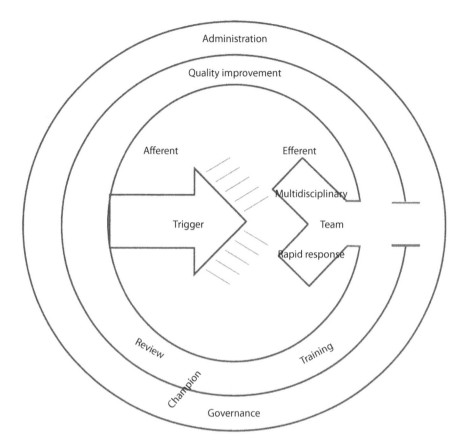

**FIGURE 2.1** Conceptual model for RRTs. (Adapted from ACOG, *Obstetrics & Gynecology*, 123, 722–725, 2014; Stolldorf, D. P. et al., Sustaining innovations in complex health care environments: A multiple-case study of rapid response teams, *Journal of Patient Safety*, 1–7, 2016; DeVita, M. A. et al., Findings of the first consensus conference on medical emergency teams, *Critical Care Medicine*, 34, 529–534, 1999; Stolldorf, D. P., and Jones, C. B., *Joint Commission Journal on Quality and Patient Safety*, 41, 186–192, 2015; Richardson, M. G. et al., *Current Opinion in Anesthesiology*, 29, 268–272, 2016.)

## REFERENCES

1. Goldhill DR, White SA, Sumner A. Physiological values and procedures in the 24h before ICU admission from the ward. *Anaesthesia*. 1999; 54:529-534.
2. DeVita MA, Bellomo R, Hillman K, Kellum J, Rotondi A, Teres D et al. Findings of the first consensus conference on medical emergency reams. *Crit Care Med*. 2006; 34:2463-2478.
3. Stolldorf DP, Jones CB. The deployment of rapid response teams in U.S. hospitals. *Jt Comm J Qual Patient Saf*. 2015; 41:186-192.
4. ACOG (American College of Obstetricians and Gynecologists) Committee on Patient Safety and Quality Improvement. ACOG Committee Opinion No. 590: Preparing for clinical emergencies in obstetrics and gynecology. *Obstet Gynecol*. 2014; 123:722-725.
5. Jones D, Rublotta F, Welch J. Rapid response teams improve outcomes: Yes. *Intensive Care Med*. 2016; 42:593-595.
6. Kimsky WS. Rapid Response Teams: Lessons from the Early Experience. *AHRQ Patient Safety Network*. 2005. Available from: https//psnet.ahrq.gov.
7. Barwise A, Thongprayoon C, Gajic O, Jensen J, Herasevich V, Pickering BW. Delayed rapid response team activation is associated with increased hospital mortality, morbidity, and length of stay in a tertiary care institution. *Crit Care Med*. 2016; 44:54-63.
8. Jones, DA, DeVita MA, Bellomo R. Rapid-response teams. *New Engl J Med*. 2011; 365:139-146.

9. Lewis G. Saving mothers' lives: Reviewing maternal deaths to make motherhood safer—2003–2005. The Seventh Report on Confidential Enquiries into Maternal Deaths in the United Kingdom. London: Confidential Enquiry into Maternal and Child Health; 2007.

10. Singh A, Guleria K, Vaid NB, Jain S. Evaluation of maternal early obstetric warning system (MEOWS chart) as a predictor of obstetric morbidity: A prospective observational study. *Eur J Obstet Gynecol Reprod Biol.* 2016; 207:11-17.

11. Singh S, McGlennan A, England A, Simons R. A validation study of the CEMACH recommended modified early obstetric warning system (MEOWS). *J Assoc Anaesth Great Br Irel.* 2012; 67:12-18.

12. Quinn AC, Meek T, Waldmann C. Obstetric early warning systems to prevent bad outcome. *Curr Opin Anesth.* 2016; 29:268-272.

13. Richardson MG, Domaradzki KA, McWeeney DT. Implementing an obstetric emergency team response system: Overcoming barriers and sustaining response dose. *Joint Comm. J Qual Patient Safety.* 2015; 41:514-521.

14. Stolldorf DP, Havens DS, Jones CB. Sustaining innovations in complex health care environments: A multiple-case study of rapid response teams. *J Patient Safety.* 2016; 1-7.

# 3

## Shock

**Arthur Jason Vaught, MD**

## CONTENTS

## Background

### Definition

Shock, or acute circulatory failure, is a life-threatening condition of imbalance of oxygen demand and supply that often leads to intensive care unit admission, multiorgan failure, and even death (see Figure 3.1). It often begins with an inciting event (infection, traumatic injury, myocardial infarction) and can eventually progress to multiorgan failure. It can be best defined as tissue hypoxia, anaerobic cellular metabolism, or inadequate oxygen utilization. Shock in itself may or may not be reversible depending on the cause and the time frame of recognition and intervention. When shock is not differentiated, it is imperative for the provider to adequately assess the patient to discern the source or reason for the cardiovascular collapse. Shock differentiation is important so that the provider can implement the correct therapies and interventions to adequately address hypotension, organ malperfusion, and, ultimately, failure.

This chapter will focus on shock as it relates to the *obstetric* provider and his or her patients. The chapter will focus on the stages of shock and its classification, how to assess shock, and how to expeditiously implement interventions to correctly reverse organ injury and hypoxia.

### Cellular Mechanism and Initial Assessment of Shock

Cellular hypoxia occurs as a result of impaired or reduced tissue oxygenation; this is secondary to either reduced oxygen-carrying capacity or delivery in the setting of increased oxygen consumption. This results in the physical characteristics of shock. Cellular hypoxia can cause intracellular edema, which, in turn, can lead to cell wall membrane pump dysfunction and leakage of intracellular contents into the extracellular space (1,2). When these biochemical processes remain unchecked, the result is acidosis,

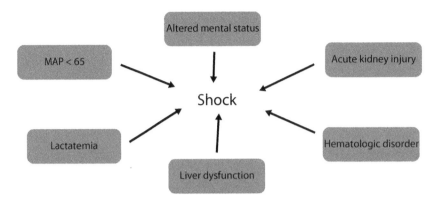

FIGURE 3.1   Signs of hypoperfusion. MAP, mean arterial pressure.

pH imbalance, release of proinflammatory cytokines that can worsen shock, and humoral processes that can impair regional blood flow (3). This microcirculatory derangement causes increased microvascular permeability, interstitial edema formation, and viscosity alterations (1,3–5).

The physiological manifestation of the shock caused by cellular damage ultimately depends on the etiology of shock itself, which will be further discussed in the next section. Although the physiological and cellular mechanism may be dissimilar, patients often have the same physical characteristics of organ failure. This includes, but is not limited to, altered mental status secondary to poor cerebral perfusion, cardiovascular hypotension from loss of preload, systemic vascular resistance or cardiac output, liver dysfunction, and renal dysfunction resulting in acute kidney injury or failure with associated anuria.

Lab values that assess tissue hypoxia can be invaluable in the initial assessment of shock. Usually, tissue hypoxia, anaerobic metabolism results in a widened anion gap acidosis secondary to lactate formation (6). Inability to clear lactate has also been observed as a marker of increased mortality in critically ill or severely injured patients (7–9). In shock, although end points of resuscitation remain controversial, lactate has been accepted as a marker of improvements in hemodynamics and prognostic outcome (9). When lactate is elevated, it should be rechecked until it returns to normal values, as patients that have improved lactate or evidence of clearance have associated improved outcomes compared to their counterparts (10). When lactate is not cleared after initial resuscitation, it should prompt the provider to consider other methods of resuscitation and evaluation. These methods could be the addition of vasopressor or ionotropic agents, blood products to increase oxygen delivery, and insertion of invasive monitors or more invasive measures such as source control in septic shock, or cardiac bypass or aortic balloon pump in cardiogenic shock.

## Classes of Shock

### Hypovolemic Shock: Hemorrhagic and Nonhemorrhagic

#### Hemorrhagic Shock

Obstetric hemorrhage accounts for 5% of all deliveries and is usually defined as >500 mL and >1000 mL of estimated blood loss following a vaginal and cesarean delivery, respectively (11). A large majority of the hemorrhages are secondary uterine atony and is resolved with medical management such as oxytocin, carboprost, and methergine (11,12). However, in patients with complex hemorrhages, which are refractory to initial management, the obstetrician must be shrewd in their management of controlled bleeding and ongoing resuscitation.

The first-line management of hemorrhagic shock, as for all shock, is the maternal ability to maintain a patent airway to aid in continuing a normal acid–base status in anaerobic metabolism (13). Afterward, a large bore venous access should be ensured. Initial fluid responsiveness is common in young healthy individuals; however, with ongoing bleeding, this could transition to blood product administration and intermittent vasopressor use.

After the stabilization of airway and venous access and ongoing fluid or blood, the third and most important step is arguably the cessation of bleeding. Generally, many obstetric hemorrhages from the uterine atony are cessated with medical therapy. However, providers may find themselves using a balloon tamponade or a uterine packing for uterine compression and decreased uterine artery perfusion (14). In the setting of maternal stability, uterine artery embolization can be pursued; however, failure rates have been recognized to be as high as 11% (15–17). Since the majority of bleeding in obstetrics is from the uterus, if hemorrhage persists, then hysterectomy is warranted, especially if there is worsening acidosis and hemodynamic instability.

While the cessation of bleeding in hemorrhage is the mainstay of therapy, one should make all attempts to avoid disseminated intravascular coagulopathy (DIC). In the setting of ongoing massive hemorrhage, many institutions have massive transfusion protocols (MTPs) to aid in resuscitation efforts. Obstetric MTP is similar to that of traumatic injury where the goal is to transfuse blood to restore oxygen-carrying capacity, while the plasma and platelets restore physiological homeostasis (18,19).

## Nonhemorrhagic Shock

Nonhemorrhagic shock is also commonly seen in maternal medicine. Patients with diabetic ketoacidosis (DKA) and hyperemesis gravidarum can have huge volume losses as a result of disease. In the setting of severe dehydration or volume loss in nonhemorrhagic shock, both physical exam and laboratory data (Table 3.1) are useful.

In DKA, there is a widened anion gap, which not only is usually secondary to serum ketones but can also be secondary to lactic acidosis. Other electrolyte abnormalities can be hyponatremia and pseudohyponatremia, hypokalemia, and hypophosphatemia (20,21). Although the mainstay of therapy is electrolyte replacement and insulin administration, fluid resuscitation is also a major intervention in DKA. In DKA, patients may have up to a 6 L total body water deficit. To help correct this deficit, one can initial start with liter boluses of (0.9% Normal Saline) for aggressive resuscitation during shock, but after the patient is hemodynamically stable, the provider can transition to isotonic saline at a rate of 15–20 mL/kg lean body weight per hour with transition to an intravenous fluid rate of 150 cc/hour (22).

Other disease states that have severe dehydration that could require aggressive crystalloid resuscitation are thyroid storm, hyperemesis gravidarum, and second- and third-degree burns.

## Distributive Shock

Distributive shock is characterized by the loss of systemic vasculature resistance and vasodilation. In maternal and obstetric care, distributive shock can be secondary to infection (septic shock), neuroaxial blockade (neurogenic shock), anaphylaxis (anaphylactic shock), and adrenal crisis (endocrine shock).

TABLE 3.1

Helpful Laboratory Investigations in Assessment of Shock

| |
|---|
| Complete blood count |
| Comprehensive metabolic panel |
| Arterial blood gas |
| Serum lactate |
| Coagulation panel including fibrinogen |
| Central venous blood gas (if central venous access available) |
|    Mixed venous oxygen saturation ($SvO_2$) |
|    Central venous oxygen saturation ($ScvO_2$) |
| Thyroid studies |

In septic shock, the mainstay is early goal-directed therapy with aggressive fluid resuscitation while avoiding fluid overload, obtaining appropriate lab and culture data, and administration of broad-spectrum antibiotics and source control (23). Although initial fluid resuscitation (30 mL/kg) is recommended by the 2013 Surviving Sepsis Guidelines, subsequent studies have shown that there is no difference in mortality between early goal and nonearly goal groups; however, in these groups, there was no statistical significance in the timing of antibiotic administration (23–25). In the setting of septic shock, norepinephrine (0.02–2 mcg/kg/minute) is the vasopressor of choice even in the pregnant population. With rising norepinephrine requirement, the provider can add vasopressin at a low dose (0.03 units/minute) (23). It should be noted that the addition of vasopressin does not change mortality, but it can help de-escalate the need for norepinephrine (26).

As stated earlier, the mainstay of therapy and distributive shock is initial fluid administration; however, the practitioner should be familiar with excessive fluid overload and the risk of pulmonary edema and abdominal compartment syndrome. Therefore, practitioners should consider vasopressor use when they feel that the patient has had adequate fluid resuscitation.

## Neurogenic Shock

Neurogenic shock is not common in maternal medicine with the exception of lumbar epidural dosing during labor and cesarean section. One of the most common complications after neuroaxial blockade is the reduction in blood pressure. Even small doses of local anesthetic (i.e., bupivacaine lidocaine) can produce a sympathetic block and cause severe hypotension (27). Because most times, this is in the setting of epidural anesthesia; it is always prudent to call for your anesthesia colleague. Generally, in neurogenic shock, the mode of therapy is combined vasopressor and fluid resuscitation until the effect of the hypotension from the local anesthetic resolves.

## Anaphylactic Shock

By far, the most common type of anaphylactic shock in pregnancy is related to amniotic fluid embolism (AFE). AFE, also called the anaphylactoid syndrome of pregnancy, is a catastrophic condition that can be described with fulminant DIC accompanied by cardiovascular collapse and respiratory failure during labor or immediately after or during delivery (28,29). The disease is rare and affects approximately 1 in 40,000 deliveries (28). It is thought that the amniotic fluid and fetal antigen enters the maternal circulation which then precipitate a massive inflammatory and anaphylactoid response (28).

The circulatory collapse of AFE is not completely clear. It is theorized to be a rapid development of pulmonary hypertension and acute cor pulmonale caused by the vasoconstrictive properties of amniotic fluid in animal models and case reports (30–32). However, some studies using invasive hemodynamic monitoring from women with AFE seem to contradict these studies, and it is suggestive that hemodynamic collapse is secondary to left ventricular failure, rather than pulmonary hypertension and right ventricular failure.

A biphasic pattern of cardiovascular collapse for AFE has been proposed recognizing that there can be both severe pulmonary hypertension and left ventricular failure. According to this hypothesis, the right ventricular failure, precedes left ventricular failure (28–30).

This type of shock can be one of the most complex types of shock to care for, mainly because it is a combination of distributive shock, cardiogenic, shock, and hemorrhagic shock secondary to DIC. First and foremost, because of the profound respiratory failure, an airway should be secured for adequate oxygenation and ventilation. At that point, there will likely need to be combined intravenous resuscitation with both crystalloid fluids along with blood products to increase the oxygen-carrying capacity while avoiding DIC. In this setting, a vasopressor will most certainly need to be used, but unlike sepsis, there is no vasopressor of choice. Because of the combined left ventricular failure, an epinephrine infusion may be of use as it has both beta and alpha adrenergic receptors, which will aid in cardiac contractility. It is likely that multiple pressors will be needed in this particular type of shock. Transthoracic and transesophageal echocardiography as well invasive monitoring such as Swan–Ganz catheter, and central venous monitoring can be extremely helpful in guiding ionotropic and vasopressor use.

## Obstructive Shock

Causes of obstructive shock can range from massive pulmonary embolism (PE), cardiac tamponade, to tension pneumothorax, to name a few. The mainstay of therapy for obstructive shock is the removal of the impedance, whether it be a chest tube for pneumothorax, pericardial drain for effusion, or embolectomy with tissue plasminogen activator (tPA) for massive PE. This requires a thorough knowledge of the patient's history and risk factors for such events such as central lines placement and lung biopsy.

In the setting of a pulmonary embolism resulting in obstructive shock, the rapid reversal of the obstruction is the primary objective. In the setting of persistent hypotension, thrombolysis with tPA is widely accepted (33). Major contraindications to the use of thrombolytics are structural intracranial disease, ischemic stroke within 3 months, active bleeding, traumatic injury, and recent neurosurgery. Pregnancy remains a relative contraindication; however, because delivery, either vaginal or cesarean, can be unpredictable, the administration of systemic tPA places the maternal patient at significant bleeding risk (33).

Successful systemic thrombolysis has been reported in pregnancy, but catheter-directed thrombolysis either with embolectomy alone or with tPA is a viable option and may reduce the risk of bleeding (34). Besides hypotension, other parameters for the need for embolectomy or thrombolysis are severe or worsening right ventricular dysfunction ("submassive pulmonary embolism"), cardiopulmonary arrest secondary to pulmonary embolism, extensive clot burden, free-floating thrombi in the right cardiac chambers, and a patent foramen ovale (35). Some patients may need surgical intervention consisting of sternotomy with rapid cannulation and cardiac bypass. Indications for surgery are patients with acute, massive PE along with contraindications to thrombolytic therapy or who have lacked a response to thrombolysis (35).

In the setting of cardiac tamponade from pericardial effusion and tension pneumothorax, clinical suspicion should be high, as usually, these patients will have risk factors (Table 3.2). Ultimately, the removal of the obstructions should be expeditiously accomplished to return perfusable blood pressure.

## Cardiogenic Shock

Cardiogenic shock is defined as anaerobic metabolism precipitated by cardiac pump failure. When the obstetric practitioner is faced with cardiac failure, it is important to categorize the reason for pump failure. Cardiac pump failure can be secondary to cardiomyopathic failure, arrhythmogenic failure (tachyarrhythmia and bradyarrhythmia), and valvular failure (i.e., critical aortic stenosis and mitral valve stenosis) (36). Although pregnant women can experience all classifications of failure, the most common associated with obstetrics will likely be cardiomyopathic failure (i.e., peripartum cardiomyopathy and myocardial infarction). Women presenting in suspected cardiogenic shock should have baseline laboratory investigations, thyroid studies, biochemical cardiac markers, electrocardiography, and echocardiogram to help differentiate etiology of failure.

The management of cardiac failure in pregnancy is very similar to that in the nonpregnant state with the goal to obtain perfusion; the etiology of pump failure helps guide therapy. In the setting of cardiac failure in pregnancy, it is helpful to establish the patient's intravascular volume status. This can be accomplished by physical exam, cardiac sonography, and invasive monitoring such as Swan–Ganz

TABLE 3.2

Risk Factors for Tension Pneumothorax and Cardiac Tamponade

| Pericardial Tamponade | Tension Pneumothorax |
| --- | --- |
| Autoimmune disease | Central line placement or lung biopsy |
|   Lupus, rheumatoid arthritis | Cystic fibrosis or other lung parenchymal diseases |
| Cancer | Traumatic injury with rib fractures |
| Renal failure with uremia | History of pneumothorax |
| Tuberculosis | Mechanical ventilation |
| Myocardial infarction | |
| Pericarditis | |

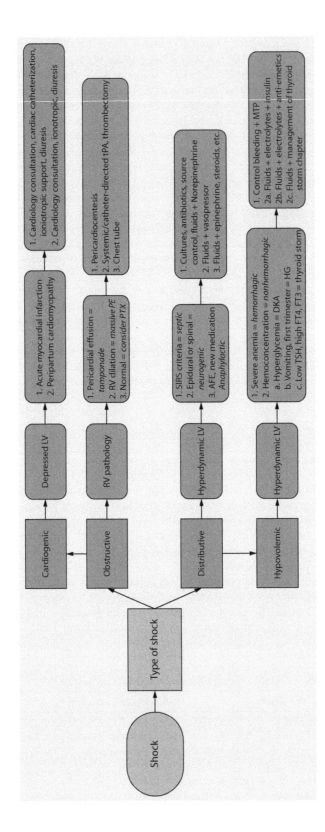

**FIGURE 3.2** Differential management of shock. FT3, Free T3; FT4, Free T4; HG, hyperemesis gravidarium; LV, left ventricle; PE, pulmonary embolism; PTX, pneumothorax; RV, right ventricle; TSH, Thyroid stimulating hormone.

catheterization. Vasopressor agents should be utilized more frequently, and intravascular volume resuscitation can be utilized, but acknowledging the risk of putting the patient into fluid overload is important.

In all, it is important to distinguish cardiogenic shock from distributive and hypovolemic shock. This can be accomplished by physical exam to look for fluid overload (i.e., jugular venous distention, pulmonary edema, pitting edema in extremities, and cool vasoconstricted extremities). Also a point of care, critical care cardiac ultrasound assesses ventricular function for severe hypokinesis.

The differential management is summarized in Figure 3.2.

## Conclusion

In any form of shock, it is important to understand the catalyst for hypoperfusion and multiorgan failure. The patient should be quickly optimized before delivery. The obstetrician should include needed intensivist, proceduralist, anesthesiologist, and subspecialist depending on shock etiology. Either way, maternal stability should be a priority and a multidisciplinary approach should be used.

## REFERENCES

1. Kristensen SR. Mechanisms of cell damage and enzyme release. *Dan Med Bull.* 1994; 41(4):423-433.
2. Barber AE, Shires GT. Cell damage after shock. *New Horiz.* 1996; 4(2):161-167.
3. Hinshaw LB. Sepsis/septic shock: Participation of the microcirculation: An abbreviated review. *Crit Care Med.* 1996; 24(6):1072-1078.
4. Chien S. Rheology in the microcirculation in normal and low flow states. *Adv Shock Res.* 1982; 8:71-80.
5. Sibbald WJ. Circulatory responses to the sepsis syndrome. *Prog Clin Biol Res.* 1989; 308:1075-1085.
6. Kreisberg RA. Lactate homeostasis and lactic acidosis. *Ann Intern Med.* 1980; 92(2 Pt 1):227-237.
7. Broder G, Weil MH. Excess lactate: An index of reversibility of shock in human patients. *Science.* 1964; 143(3613):1457-1459.
8. Mikkelsen ME, Miltiades AN, Gaieski DF, Goyal M, Fuchs B, Shah CV et al. Serum lactate is associated with mortality in severe sepsis independent of organ failure and shock. *Crit Care Med.* 2009; 37(5):1670-1677.
9. Abramson D, Scalea TM, Hitchcock R, Trooskin SZ, Henry SM, Greenspan J. Lactate clearance and survival following injury. *J Trauma.* 1993; 35(4):584-588.
10. Nguyen HB, Rivers EP, Knoblich BP, Jacobsen G, Muzzin A, Ressler JA et al. Early lactate clearance is associated with improved outcome in severe sepsis and septic shock. *Crit Care Med.* 2004; 32(8):1637-1642.
11. Lu MC, Fridman M, Korst LM, Gregory KD, Reyes C, Hobel CJ et al. Variations in the incidence of postpartum hemorrhage across hospitals in California. *Matern Child Health J.* 2005; 9(3):297-306.
12. Sheiner E, Sarid L, Levy A, Seidman DS, Hallak M. Obstetric risk factors and outcome of pregnancies complicated with early postpartum hemorrhage: A population-based study. *J Matern Fetal Neonatal Med.* 2005; 18(3):149-154.
13. American College of Surgeons Committee on Tauma. *Advanced trauma life support: Student course manual.* 8th ed. Chicago, IL: Third Impression; 2008.
14. Belfort MA, Dildy GA, Garrido J, White GL. Intraluminal pressure in a uterine tamponade balloon is curvilinearly related to the volume of fluid infused. *Am J Perinatol.* 2011; 28(8):659-666.
15. Bros S, Chabrot P, Kastler A, Ouchchane L, Cassagnes L, Gallot D et al. Recurrent bleeding within 24 hours after uterine artery embolization for severe postpartum hemorrhage: Are there predictive factors? *Cardiovasc Intervent Radiol.* 2012; 35(3):508-514.
16. Poujade O, Zappa M, Letendre I, Ceccaldi PF, Vilgrain V, Luton D. Predictive factors for failure of pelvic arterial embolization for postpartum hemorrhage. *Int J Gynaecol Obstet.* 2012; 117(2):119-123.
17. Sentilhes L, Gromez A, Clavier E, Resch B, Verspyck E, Marpeau L. Predictors of failed pelvic arterial embolization for severe postpartum hemorrhage. *Obstet Gynecol.* 2009; 113(5):992-999.
18. Burtelow M, Riley E, Druzin M, Fontaine M, Viele M, Goodnough LT. How we treat: Management of life-threatening primary postpartum hemorrhage with a standardized massive transfusion protocol. *Transfusion.* 2007; 47(9):1564-1572.

19. Malone DL, Hess JR, Fingerhut A. Massive transfusion practices around the globe and a suggestion for a common massive transfusion protocol. *J Trauma.* 2006; 60(6 Suppl):S91-S96.
20. Abramson E, Arky R. Diabetic acidosis with initial hypokalemia: Therapeutic implications. *JAMA.* 1966; 196(5):401-403.
21. Hillier TA, Abbott RD, Barrett EJ. Hyponatremia: Evaluating the correction factor for hyperglycemia. *Am J Med.* 1999; 106(4):399-403.
22. Kitabchi AE, Umpierrez GE, Miles JM, Fisher JN. Hyperglycemic crises in adult patients with diabetes. *Diabetes Care.* 2009; 32(7):1335-1343.
23. Dellinger RP, Levy MM, Rhodes A, Annane D, Gerlach H, Opal SM et al. Surviving sepsis campaign: International guidelines for management of severe sepsis and septic shock: 2012. *Crit Care Med.* 2013; 41(2):580-637.
24. ARISE Investigators, ANZICS Clinical Trials Group. Goal-directed resuscitation for patients with early septic shock. *N Engl J Med.* 2014; 371(16):1496-1506.
25. ProCESS Investigators. A randomized trial of protocol-based care for early septic shock. *N Engl J Med.* 2014; 370(18):1683-1693.
26. Russell JA, Walley KR, Singer J, Gordon AC, Hébert PC, Cooper J et al. Vasopressin versus norepinephrine infusion in patients with septic shock. *N Engl J Med.* 2008; 358(9):877-887.
27. Eisenach JC. Combined spinal-epidural analgesia in obstetrics. *Anesthesiology.* 1999; 91(1):299-302.
28. Clark SL. Amniotic fluid embolism. *Obstet Gynecol.* 2014; 123(2 Pt 1):337-348.
29. Gilmore DA, Wakim J, Secrest J, Rawson R. Anaphylactoid syndrome of pregnancy: A review of the literature with latest management and outcome data. *AANA J.* 2003; 71(2):120-126.
30. Attwood HD, Downing ES. Experimental amniotic fluid and meconium embolism. *Surg Gynecol Obstet.* 1965; 120:255-262.
31. Shechtman M, Ziser A, Markovits R, Rozenberg B. Amniotic fluid embolism: Early findings of transesophageal echocardiography. *Anesth Analg.* 1999; 89(6):1456-1458.
32. Stanten RD, Iverson LI, Daugharty TM, Lovett SM, Terry C, Blumenstock E. Amniotic fluid embolism causing catastrophic pulmonary vasoconstriction: Diagnosis by transesophageal echocardiogram and treatment by cardiopulmonary bypass. *Obstet Gynecol.* 2003; 102(3):496-498.
33. Kearon C, Akl EA, Ornelas J, Blaivas A, Jimenez D, Bounameaux H et al. Antithrombotic therapy for VTE disease: CHEST guideline and expert panel report. *Chest.* 2016; 149(2):315-352.
34. O'Keeffe SA, McGrath A, Ryan JM, Byrne B. Management of a massive pulmonary embolism in a pregnant patient with mechanical fragmentation followed by delayed catheter-directed thrombolysis in the early postpartum period. *J Matern Fetal Neonatal Med.* 2008; 21(8):591-594.
35. Torbicki A, van Beek EJR et al. Guidelines on diagnosis and management of acute pulmonary embolism: Task force on pulmonary embolism. *Eur Heart J.* 2000; 21(16):1301-1336.
36. Califf RM, Bengtson JR. Cardiogenic shock. *N Engl J Med.* 1994; 330(24):1724-1730.

# 4

## _Severe Hypertension_

**Daniel W. Skupski, MD and Sandra Asanjarani, RNC, MS, NP**

### CONTENTS

### Introduction

A pregnant woman who experiences severe hypertension is at increased risk of serious morbidity, including abruptio placentae, hypertensive encephalopathy, acute kidney injury, and cerebrovascular accident (1,2). There is a significant long-term morbidity from these events, which justifies efforts at prevention (3).

Indeed, the incidence of stroke associated with pregnancy has increased in the United States in recent years, showing a 47% increase in stroke associated with pregnancy and an 83% increase in postpartum stroke (4,5). There are undoubtedly many factors that have contributed to this increase, including the increases in maternal age, obesity, and multifetal pregnancies due to assisted reproductive techniques (6,7). An additional factor that is not well characterized may be the increased use of nonsteroidal antiinflammatory drugs for pain control in the postpartum time period.

Recent efforts have addressed a method for lowering the risk of morbidity by treating severe hypertension more quickly than has been done previously (8) (Box 4.1). This involves protocols for antihypertensive medications to be given within a short time frame, whenever persistent severe hypertension is identified, and includes pregnant women and women up to 6 weeks postpartum (9,10). Although the vast majority of episodes of severe hypertension that present postpartum do so within 2 weeks, it is remotely possible for some to present in this fashion up to 6 weeks after delivery.

This chapter will describe the identification and treatment of acute severe hypertension and persistent severe hypertension related to pregnancy, primarily with the use of algorithms and tables that can be made available at the sites where these women are cared for—the emergency department (ED), the labor and delivery suite, and hospital wards.

### Hypertension: Technical Aspects

A classification of hypertensive disorders of pregnancy is shown in Table 4.1. Any hypertensive disorder, including preexisting chronic hypertension, may lead to antepartum, intrapartum, or postpartum acute severe hypertension (Box 4.2).

## BOX 4.1   SEVERE HYPERTENSION IN PREGNANCY

| What We Know | What We Do Not Know | What to Do |
|---|---|---|
| Severe hypertension leads to morbidity and mortality. | Which factors that contribute to the development of hypertension are the most important? | Treat promptly to decrease BP and lower risk. |

### TABLE 4.1

Classification of Hypertensive Disorders of Pregnancy

| Type of Hypertensive Disorder | Definition |
|---|---|
| Chronic hypertension | Systolic BP ≥ 140 *or* diastolic BP ≥ 90 prior to pregnancy or before 20 weeks of gestation |
| Gestational hypertension | Systolic BP ≥ 140 *or* diastolic BP ≥ 90 after 20 weeks of gestation with the absence of proteinuria and the absence of signs and symptoms of preeclampsia |
| Preeclampsia | 1. Systolic BP ≥ 140 *or* diastolic BP ≥ 90 with proteinuria *or* <br> 2. Systolic BP ≥ 140 *or* diastolic BP ≥ 90 without proteinuria with symptoms[a] *or* <br> 3. Systolic BP ≥ 140 *or* diastolic BP ≥ 90 without proteinuria with laboratory abnormalities[a] |
| Eclampsia | Seizure(s) in the setting of preeclampsia |
| Chronic hypertension with superimposed preeclampsia | Systolic BP ≥ 140 *or* diastolic BP ≥ 90 prior to pregnancy or before 20 weeks of gestation combined with new onset proteinuria, symptoms[a] or laboratory abnormalities[a] |
| Acute severe hypertension | Systolic BP ≥ 160 mmHg *or* diastolic BP ≥ 110 at any time during pregnancy or postpartum period |
| Persistent severe hypertension | Two severe BP values ≥ 160 mmHg systolic or BP ≥ 110 diastolic taken 15–60 minutes apart any time during pregnancy or the postpartum period. Severe values do not need to be consecutive |

[a]  Symptoms and laboratory abnormalities of preeclampsia with severe features are listed in Table 4.2.

## BOX 4.2   CLASSIFICATION OF HYPERTENSIVE DISORDERS OF PREGNANCY

| What We Know | What We Do Not Know | What to Do |
|---|---|---|
| • Both preexisting hypertension and pregnancy-related hypertension can lead to acute severe hypertension. <br> • BP above 130/80 in early pregnancy (<20 weeks) is distinctly abnormal. | How do we predict when, during pregnancy, BP will become severely elevated? | Use available clinical classification systems which help to define risks. |

The measurement of blood pressure (BP) has a long history (12,13). The preferred method for measuring BP during pregnancy is in the sitting position, with both feet resting on the floor, after 10 minutes of rest, with the cuff at the level of the heart. At least two values should be taken at least 1 minute apart. These values should be averaged (12). Therapy should not be decided upon on the basis of one BP alone. The sitting position is preferred because this avoids the alteration of BP that occurs during pregnancy in the supine position and the alteration of BP in the lateral recumbent position (12). At the extremes of human size (obese patients and children), the proper cuff size is also of critical importance (12).

**BOX 4.3   MEASUREMENT OF BP**

| What We Know | What We Do Not Know | What to Do |
| --- | --- | --- |
| • BP can be accurately measured by many devices. <br>• Any single BP value can be inaccurate. | • What BP patterns (diurnal variation, short-term variability, perhaps others) contribute to morbidity and mortality? <br>• What is the duration of severe hypertension at which morbidity and mortality are increased? | • Aneroid and hybrid devices require frequent calibration (11). <br>• Always take multiple BP measurements before beginning antihypertensive therapy. <br>• Treat acute severe hypertension promptly. |

There is also a long history and many publications devoted to the issue of which the method is more accurate—manual (mercury sphygmomanometer with the use of first and fifth Korotkoff sounds using a stethoscope) or automated (aneroid or hybrid devices). With either method, accuracy is reasonable (Box 4.3) (11,12,14). Aneroid and hybrid devices for measuring BP are pervasive in many inpatient and outpatient settings and are probably accurate enough to allow screening for hypertension that requires further evaluation. These devices measure mean BP and calculate systolic and diastolic pressures via the use of proprietary algorithms and, thus, probably have inferior accuracy compared to the mercury sphygmomanometer (manual device with a stethoscope). There are few devices validated for use in pregnancy (15,16).

One of the most important aspects of the measurement of BP is that the provider who measures BP and finds persistent severe hypertension communicates this finding to the treatment team. This is generally a nurse who must notify the obstetric resident or attending physician. Standard practices at all institutions should include the notification of the responsible physician in a timely manner so that antihypertensive medication can be ordered and promptly administered.

## Presentation

Common presentations include the following:

1. A second or third trimester pregnant woman with or without symptoms, who presents for a routine prenatal visit or appears in the ED, and is discovered to have acute severe hypertension
2. A woman in the postpartum time period with or without symptoms, who presents for a routine postpartum follow up visit or appears in the ED and is discovered to have acute severe hypertension

**BOX 4.4   PRESENTATION**

| What We Know | What We Do Not Know | What to Do |
| --- | --- | --- |
| • During pregnancy and up to 6 weeks postpartum, women can present with acute severe hypertension, and their risk of morbidity and mortality are increased. <br>• Symptoms of severe headache, persistent vomiting, scotomata and epigastric, or upper abdominal pain can be the only warning signs. | Why does the disease of preeclampsia present days or weeks after delivery? | • Schedule follow-up visits within 1 week of delivery for all women with hypertensive disorders of pregnancy. <br>• Educate all women about symptoms of acute severe hypertension and instruct them to seek care immediately if these occur. |

Due to the common presentation of these women in the outpatient facilities and the ED, it is important for the providers in these locations to be educated about the importance of prompt evaluation and treatment of persistent severe hypertension (Box 4.4).

## Diagnosis

Some classifications of hypertensive disorders in pregnancy have deemphasized the importance of proteinuria (3). This is due to the fact that not all patients present with the same signs and symptoms nor with the same laboratory abnormalities, because the disease does not affect all organs to an equal degree. Indeed, preeclampsia can be characterized as affecting primarily *one* organ—the vascular endothelium. Physiological derangements can occur at any organ level and can present as the signs and symptoms of "preeclampsia with severe features" (Table 4.2). The risk of morbidity when a patient presents with preeclampsia with severe features is primarily determined by whether or not there is persistent severe hypertension (2). The symptoms and laboratory abnormalities that indicate the presence of preeclampsia with severe features are shown in Table 4.3.

Acute severe hypertension can occur in the antepartum, intrapartum, and postpartum time periods. The definition of acute severe hypertension is any one of the following: mean arterial pressure (MAP) ≥130 mmHg, systolic BP ≥160 mmHg, and diastolic BP ≥110 mmHg (Table 4.3) (15,17).

If severe hypertension is detected, repeat BP measurements should be taken. See the diagnostic algorithm in Figure 4.1. If systolic BP is ≥160 *or* diastolic BP is ≥110, BP measurements should be repeated every 5 minutes for 15 minutes. If two severe values are taken 15–60 minutes apart, not necessarily consecutively, antihypertensive therapy should begin preferably within about 1 hour of the second elevated value. Persistent severe hypertension can cause cerebral hemorrhage, cerebral infarction, or hypertensive encephalopathy (18). Thus, if two BP measurements in the severe range are obtained within 15–60 minutes, treatment should be initiated.

TABLE 4.2

Severe Features of Preeclampsia

| |
|---|
| • Two values of systolic BP ≥ 160 or diastolic BP ≥ 110 obtained 4 hours apart |
| • Progressive renal insufficiency—serum creatinine ≥ 1.1 mg/dL or doubling of baseline serum creatinine |
| • Persistent severe headache |
| • New onset visual disturbances (visual blind spots or persistent blurry vision) |
| • Pulmonary edema |
| • Ascites |
| • Severe, persistent right upper quadrant or epigastric abdominal pain |
| • Liver function test (AST, ALT) abnormalities ≥ twice the upper limit of normal |
| • Platelet count less than 100,000/μL |
| • HELLP syndrome (hemolysis, elevated liver enzymes, and low Platelet count) |

*Source:*   American College of Obstetricians and Gynecologists; Executive Summary: Hypertension in Pregnancy, *Obstetrics Gynecology*, 122, 1122–1131, 2013.

*Note:*   Any one of these allows the diagnosis of preeclampsia with severe features. ALT, alanine aminotransferase; AST, aspartate aminotransferase.

TABLE 4.3

Acute Severe Hypertension and Persistent Severe Hypertension

| |
|---|
| *Acute severe hypertension*—Systolic BP ≥ 160 mmHg *or* diastolic BP ≥ 110. |
| *Persistent severe hypertension*—Two or more severe BP values taken 15–60 minutes apart. Systolic BP ≥ 160 mmHg *or* diastolic BP ≥ 110. Severe values do not need to be consecutive. |
| Persistent severe hypertension (more than one measurement) denotes an increased risk of morbidity. This can occur anytime during pregnancy, the intrapartum period, or the postpartum period. |

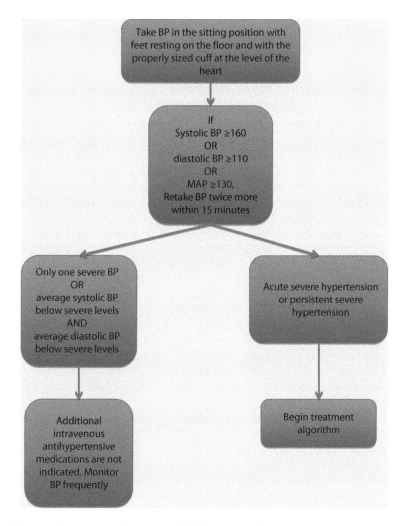

FIGURE 4.1  Diagnosis of acute severe hypertension. MAP, mean arterial pressure.

In order to reduce maternal and fetal adverse outcomes, it is imperative that prompt treatment is initiated, the need for seizure prophylaxis is determined and provided if necessary, and a decision is made about the timing of delivery.

## Treatment

In the nonpregnant patient, the goals for treating BP are to bring the diastolic BP below 90 for the younger patient (aged 30–59) and to bring BP below 150/90 in the older patient (aged 60 and above) (19). If the patient is pregnant, the goal of the treatment is not to normalize BP, but to achieve a BP range of 140–159 mmHg systolic and 90–109 mmHg diastolic in order to prevent repeated prolonged exposure of the patient to severe systolic hypertension, with subsequent loss of cerebral autoregulation (3). The loss of cerebral autoregulation is the key event in the production of intracranial hemorrhage and hypertensive encephalopathy (20). Because morbidity is primarily related to persistent severe hypertension, BP should be promptly treated (Box 4.5). If a decision is made for cesarean delivery, intubation and general anesthesia can increase BP, sometimes to dangerous levels. BP should be stabilized first (if possible in the time allowed) in order to minimize the hypertensive response to induction anesthesia. In the setting of extreme elevations of BP, such as ≥200/120, the aim is generally to lower BP by no more than

**BOX 4.5 TREATMENT**

| What We Know | What We Do Not Know | What to Do |
|---|---|---|
| When acute severe hypertension is present, lowering BP decreases morbidity and mortality. | Which medication is the best initial treatment for acute severe hypertension in pregnancy and postpartum? | Treat acute severe hypertension promptly. |

25% per hour in an effort to allow the continuation of adequate cerebral perfusion (21). If the patient is postpartum, BP target levels can be lower (90 mmHg or lower diastolic BP) because the higher pressure levels needed to provide better uteroplacental blood flow and oxygenation to the fetus are no longer necessary. A treatment algorithm is seen in Figure 4.2.

The preferred agents for antihypertensive therapy for persistent severe hypertension related to pregnancy are listed in Table 4.4 (22). Labetalol and hydralazine are preferred intravenous (IV) agents because of their rapid onset of action. If IV access has not yet been established, orally administered nifedipine is also acceptable, but establishing IV access is of primary importance. If BP remains severely elevated despite the initial dose of antihypertensive medication, additional doses should be provided as frequently as necessary according to the algorithm in Figure 4.2. If BP cannot be controlled after reaching the end of the algorithm, critical care consultation is prudent. Additional medications that may help in lowering BP are nitroprusside, nicardipine, and fenoldopam (21,23,24).

The need for seizure prophylaxis should be assessed. If eclampsia is present or signs or symptoms of preeclampsia with severe features are present, magnesium sulfate seizure prophylaxis is clearly superior to other antiseizure medications (Table 4.5) (22,25–28). In addition, seizure prophylaxis is indicated if the following are present: unilateral or localizing neurologic signs, hyperreflexia, and mental status changes. In essence, it may be prudent to provide magnesium sulfate seizure prophylaxis for any worsening sign or symptom relating to neurologic status. Seizure prophylaxis with magnesium sulfate is generally provided for 12–24 hours, or, if the patient is still pregnant, until 24 hours after delivery. For the patient who presents postpartum, the algorithms for diagnosis and management are the same, although there does not need to be an evaluation of the fetus. (See Chapter 10 for management of seizures.)

Once BP is controlled (<160/110), frequent reevaluation is necessary. A common practice is to measure BP every 10 minutes for 1 hour, every 15 minutes for the next hour, every 30 minutes for the next hour, and every hour for the following 4 hours. Laboratory tests that should be obtained and followed are complete blood count (including platelet count), lactate dehydrogenase, liver function tests (aspartate aminotransferase [AST], alanine aminotransferase [ALT], and bilirubin), electrolytes, blood urea nitrogen, creatinine, and urine protein (24-hour urine protein measurement or urine protein/creatinine ratio).

## Subsequent Management

For the pregnant patient with preeclampsia, stabilization with rest in a hospital over many days or weeks after the acute episode of severe hypertension is prudent. Delivery is not always immediately necessary. It is possible, indeed common, to delay delivery for days or weeks with the practice of rest in the hospital. A switch to oral antihypertensive medications may be appropriate, particularly in women with chronic hypertension.

In the postpartum time frame, oral antihypertensive medications are not always necessary, and if medications are provided upon discharge, it should be remembered that BP levels may decrease as the disease process resolves over the following few days or more. It is important to have all women who experienced gestational hypertension or preeclampsia return for evaluation and BP check in 1 week or less after discharge. BP levels may decrease such that antihypertensive medications can be discontinued. Alternatively, the recruitment of extravascular fluid into the vascular space can lead to high-volume hypertension between the third and seventh postpartum days and subsequent acute severe hypertension.

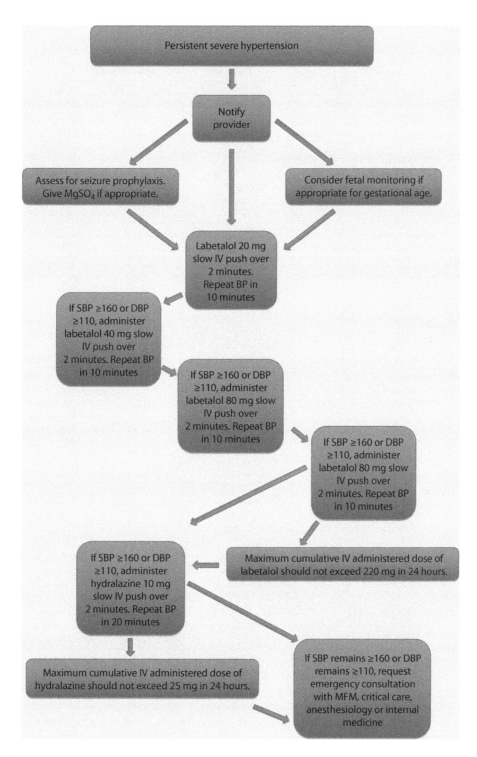

**FIGURE 4.2** Management of persistent severe hypertension. Superiority of any one medication as the initial choice has not been demonstrated. The choice of labetalol first is a common practice (SBP, systolic blood pressure; DBP, diastolic blood pressure; MFM, maternal fetal medicine).

TABLE 4.4

Preferred Agents for Antihypertensive Therapy for Persistent Severe Hypertension in Obstetrics

| Agent | Route | Dose | Frequency | Maximum Amount | Comment |
|-------|-------|------|-----------|----------------|---------|
| Labetalol[a] | IV slowly over 2 minutes | 20 mg, then 40 mg, then 80 mg, then 80 mg | Every 10 minutes | 220 mg in 24 hours | Avoid with maternal bradycardia, symptomatic asthma and asthma currently being treated |
| Hydralazine | IV slowly over 2 minutes | 5 mg, then 10 mg, then 10 mg | Every 20 minutes | 25 mg in 24 hours | Avoid with maternal tachycardia |
| Nifedipine[b] | Oral | 10 mg, then 20 mg, then 20 mg | Every 30 minutes | 50 mg in 1 hour | *Not* extended release formulation; oral, *not* sublingual |

[a] If the heart rate is below 60 beats per minute, hold labetalol or switch to another medication. Labetalol at high doses is rarely associated with hypokalemia, which would mandate the discontinuation of labetalol and the need for cardiac telemetry.

[b] Rare synergism of nifedipine with $MgSO_4$ may lead to hypotension and mandate the discontinuation of $MgSO_4$.

TABLE 4.5

Seizure Prophylaxis

| Agent | Bolus Dose and Route | Maintenance Dose and Route | Maintenance Frequency | Comment |
|-------|----------------------|----------------------------|-----------------------|---------|
| Magnesium sulfate[a] | 4–6 g IV over 20 minutes | 1–2 g IV | Every hour | 6 g bolus is recommended to mimic the original pharmacokinetics of IM administration originally proposed by Pritchard (26) and Pritchard et al. (27) |
| | 5 g of 50% solution intramuscular (IM) in each buttock (two injections simultaneously) | 5 g IM | Every 4 hours | |
| Lorazepam (Ativan) | 2–4 mg IV | May be repeated once after 10–15 minutes if seizures continue | – | |
| Diazepam (Valium) | 5–10 mg IV | 5–10 mg IV every 5–10 minutes, maximum of dose 30 mg | | |
| Phenytoin (Dilantin) | 15–20 mg/kg IV | May be repeated once 10 mg/kg IV after 20 minutes if seizures continue | – | Avoid with hypotension; may cause cardiac arrhythmias |
| Levetiracetam (Keppra) | 500 mg IV or oral | May repeat 500 mg IV or oral in 12 hours | – | Dose adjustment is needed if renal impairment is present |

[a] If renal failure or acute kidney injury is present, the 4–6 g loading dose will provide the levels of $MgSO_4$ necessary for anticonvulsant prevention and the maintenance dose should *not* be given.

There are unusual cases of women without gestational hypertension or preeclampsia before delivery who return to the ED with acute severe hypertension (Box 4.6). The diagnostic and management principles outlined here also apply to these women.

## Summary

The increased risk of morbidity and mortality with hypertensive emergencies mandates a prompt and coordinated approach to management, which includes the serial assessment of BP, close monitoring,

**BOX 4.6   SUBSEQUENT MANAGEMENT**

| What We Know | What We Do Not Know | What to Do |
|---|---|---|
| Long-term treatment of hypertension (>140/90) lowers morbidity. | Which oral medications are optimal during the postpartum time period? | Use oral medications that are effective and safe for breastfeeding. |

antihypertensive treatment with (usually IV) medications, seizure prophylaxis, and the involvement of experienced physicians. The charts and algorithms provided in this chapter can be used to highlight an approach for management in any of the sites where such patients present.

# REFERENCES

1. Russo CA, Andrews RM. *Hospital stays for stroke and other cerebrovascular diseases, 2005.* HCUP Statistical Brief No. 51. Rockville, MD: Agency for Healthcare Research and Quality; 2008.
2. Buchbinder A, Sibai BM, Caritis S MacPherson C, Hauth J, Lindheimer MD et al. Adverse perinatal outcomes are significantly higher in severe gestational hypertension than in mild preeclampsia. *Am J Obstet Gynecol.* 2002; 186:66-71.
3. American College of Obstetricians and Gynecologists. Executive summary: Hypertension in pregnancy. *Obstet Gynecol.* 2013; 122:1122-1131.
4. Kuklina EV, Tong X, Bansil P, George MG, Callaghan WM. Trends in pregnancy hospitalizations that included a stroke in the United States from 1994 to 2007: Reasons for concern? *Stroke.* 2011; 42:2564-2570.
5. Kuklina EV, Ayala C, Callaghan WM. Hypertensive disorders and severe obstetric morbidity in the United States. *Obstet Gynecol.* 2009; 113:1299-1306.
6. Ogden CL, Carroll MD, Curtin LR, McDowell MA, Tabak CJ, Flegal KM. Prevalence of overweight and obesity in the United States, 1999-2004. *J Am Med Assoc.* 2006; 295:1549-1555.
7. Heron M, Sutton, PD, Xu J, Ventura SJ, Strobino DM, Guyer B. Annual summary of vital statistics: 2007. *Pediatrics.* 2010; 125:4-15.
8. Burgansky A, MontaltoD, Siddiqui NA. The safe motherhood initiative: The development and implementation of standardized obstetric care bundles in New York. *Semin Perinatol.* 2016 Mar; 40(2):124-131.
9. Moroz LA, Simpson LL, Rochelson B. Management of severe hypertension in pregnancy. *Semin Perinatol.* 2016; 40(2):112-118.
10. Martin JN. Severe systolic hypertension and the search for safer motherhood. *Semin Perinatol.* 2016; 40(2):119-123.
11. O'Brien E, Pickering T, Asmar R, Myers M, Parati G, Staessen J et al. Working group on blood pressure monitoring of the European Society of Hypertension International Protocol for validation of blood pressure measuring devices in adults. *Blood Press Monit.* 2002; 7:3-17.
12. Pickering TG, Hall JE, Appel LJ, Falkner BE, Graves J, Hill MN et al. Recommendations for blood pressure measurement in humans and animals: Part 1: Blood pressure measurement in humans: A statement for professionals from the Subcommittee of Professional and Public Education of the American Heart Association Council on High Blood Pressure Research. *Hypertension.* 2005; 45:142-161.
13. Ogedegbe G, Pickering T. Principles and techniques of blood pressure measurement. *Cardiol. Clin.* 2010; 28:571-586.
14. Natarajan P, Shennan A, Penny J, Halligan A, de Swiet M, Anthony J. Comparison of auscultatory and oscillometric automated blood pressure monitors in the setting of preeclampsia. *Am J Obstet Gynecol.* 1999; 181:1203-1210.
15. Brown MA, Davis GK. Hypertension in pregnancy. In: Mancia G, Chalmers J, Julius S, Saruta T, Weber MA Ferrari AU et al., editors. *Manual of hypertension.* London: Harcourt Publishers; 2002, pp. 579-597.
16. Golara M, Benedict A, Jones C, Randhawa M, Poston L, Shennan AH. Inflationary oscillometry provides accurate measurement of blood pressure in pre-eclampsia. *BJOG.* 2002 Oct; 109(10):1143-1147.

17. Brown MA, Lindheimer MD, de Swiet M, Van Assche A, Moutquin JM. The classification and diagnosis of the hypertensive disorders of pregnancy: Statement from the International Society for the Study of Hypertension in Pregnancy (ISSHP). *Hypertens Pregnancy.* 2001; 20(1):IX-XIV.

18. Martin JN, Thigpen BD, Moore RC, Rose CH, Cushman J, May W. Stroke and severe preeclampsia and eclampsia: A paradigm shift focusing on systolic blood pressure. *Obstet Gynecol.* 2005; 105:246-254.

19. Chobanian AV, Bakris GL, Black HR, Cushman WC, Green LA, Izzo Jr JL et al. The seventh report of the Joint National Committee on Prevention, Detection, Evaluation and Treatment of High Blood Pressure: The JNC 7 report. *JAMA.* 2003; 289:2560-2572.

20. Kilpatrick SJ, Abreo A, Greene N, Melsop K, Peterson N, Shields LE et al. Severe maternal morbidity in a large cohort of women with acute severe intrapartum hypertension. *Am J Obstet Gynecol.* 2016; 215:91.e1-e7.

21. Vaughan CJ, Delanty N. Hypertensive emergencies. *Lancet.* 2000; 356:411-417.

22. Barton JR, Sibai BM. Management of hypertensive crisis including stroke. In Sibai MB, editor. *Management of acute obstetric emergencies.* Philadelphia, PA: Elsevier Saunders; 2011, pp. 101-113.

23. Padilla Ramos A, Varon J. Current and newer agents for hypertensive emergencies. *Curr Hypertens Rep.* 2014; 16:450.

24. Mancia G, Fagard R, Narkiewicz K, Redon J, Zanchetti A, Böhm M et al. 2013 ESH/ESC guidelines for the management of arterial hypertension: The Task Force for the management of arterial hypertension of the European Society of Hypertension (ESH) and of the European Society of Cardiology (ESC). *J Hypertens.* 2013; 31:1281-1357.

25. James PA, Oparil S, Carter BL, Cushman WC, Dennison-Himmelfarb C, Handler J et al. 2014 Evidence-based guideline for the management of high blood pressure in adults report from the panel members appointed to the Eighth Joint National Committee (JNC 8). *JAMA.* 2014; 311(5):507-520.

26. Pritchard JA. The use of magnesium ion in the management of eclamptogenic toxemias. *Surg Gynecol Obstet.* 1955; 100:131-140.

27. Pritchard JA, Cunningham FG, Pritchard SA. The Parkland Memorial Hospital protocol for treatment of eclampsia: Evaluation of 245 cases. *Am J Obstet Gynecol.* 1984; 148:951-963.

28. Lucas MJ, Leveno KJ, Cunningham FG. A comparison of magnesium sulfate with phenytoin for the prevention of eclampsia. *New Engl J Med.* 1995; 333:201-205.

# 5

## Arrhythmia

**Melissa Westermann, MD and Afshan B. Hameed, MD, FACC, FACOG**

### CONTENTS

## Introduction

Palpitations—"awareness of the heartbeat"—are the most common cardiac-related complaint in general, and arrhythmias are one of the most frequently encountered cardiac diagnoses in pregnancy. Typically, arrhythmias are due to a preexisting cardiac disease; however, it is not uncommon to see new-onset arrhythmias in women without evidence of a structural cardiac defect (1–3). Pregnancy by virtue of its hormonal milieu may aggravate previously well-controlled arrhythmias or may unmask an undiagnosed cardiac condition, with arrhythmia being the initial/presenting manifestation (4–6). The exact etiology of the de novo arrhythmia in pregnancy is unclear; however, it is likely based on the hemodynamic, hormonal, and autonomic alterations of pregnancy (7).

Maternal cardiovascular system adapts to the growing metabolic requirements of pregnancy by virtue of several hemodynamic changes. Some of these adaptations include increases in heart rate, stroke volume, and cardiac output; expansion of intravascular volume; a decreased peripheral vascular resistance; and an increase in sympathetic activity (8). A combination of these factors creates a milieu for not only initiating but also sustaining cardiac dysrhythmias during pregnancy. This is further enhanced by the heightened emotional state and visceral awareness of pregnancy that may lead women to seek advice for symptoms that otherwise would potentially be ignored. Even though the majority of arrhythmias occurring in pregnancy are benign, they do create significant anxiety and may be a source of maternal morbidity and even mortality.

## Incidence

Cardiac arrhythmias are seen in 60% of healthy young individuals on 24-hour ambulatory monitor (9). Outside of pregnancy, palpitations account for 16% of the outpatient medical visits (10). During pregnancy, only 10% of symptomatic episodes of palpitations are due to an arrhythmia (3). The event rate of arrhythmias in pregnancy, based on pregnancy-related admissions, is estimated at 166/100,000 (11). Pregnancy has a propensity to cause tachycardia; however, bradycardia may also be rarely seen. Arrhythmias range from premature atrial or ventricular contractions, supraventricular tachycardia (SVT), and atrial fibrillation to life-threatening ventricular tachycardia (VT) (3); bradycardia, on the other hand, is a relatively uncommon occurrence (1%) in pregnant women with cardiac complaints. Women with structural heart disease are at a particularly high risk of developing an arrhythmia, and arrhythmia is a strong predictor of a serious cardiac event. Highest-risk women include those with congenital heart disease (CHD) and with multiple cardiac risk factors. Advancements in the surgical and medical management of children with CHD allow them to reach reproductive years with a limited ability to withstand the hemodynamic challenge of pregnancy. Delayed childbearing and assisted reproductive technology are also enabling older women with preexisting cardiac risk factors to become pregnant, and a combination of these factors culminates into heart disease and arrhythmias increasingly seen during pregnancy (12,13).

## Diagnostic Evaluation

The key components of diagnosing an arrhythmia during pregnancy are to accurately identify the type of arrhythmia and exclude temporary or permanent exacerbating factors, systemic disorders, and/or associated structural heart disease. Typically, palpitations are considered benign in the absence of structural heart defect and are most often self-limited and resolve in the postpartum period. On the other hand, palpitations may be the first presenting symptoms of an underlying serious cardiac disease or may represent a life-threatening arrhythmia. A patient presenting with symptoms of palpitations along with dizziness or near syncope is highly suggestive of an underlying arrhythmia/heart disease and warrants further evaluation (Figure 5.1).

The diagnostic evaluation of pregnant women for an arrhythmia is similar to that of the general population. Evaluation includes a complete history, physical examination, and 12-lead electrocardiogram (ECG) ± transthoracic echocardiogram to assess cardiac structure and function. Laboratory testing includes complete blood count and thyroid function to rule out significant anemia and thyrotoxicosis, respectively. *A combination of history and physical examination, ECG, and limited laboratory testing allows a specific diagnosis in about one-third of the patients* (14). The most common cause of palpitations is cardiac (43%), followed by psychiatric (31%) illness such as anxiety, and 10% are due to medications or other causes (15). Other conditions that may cause the symptoms of an arrhythmia include mitral valve prolapse, vasovagal syncope, anxiety, hypoglycemia, heart failure, pericarditis, electrolyte imbalance, pulmonary embolism, infection, and hemorrhage. After excluding these conditions, diagnosis may ultimately be attributed to normal physiological changes in pregnancy.

A major limitation of an ECG in diagnosing arrhythmia is that symptoms are typically intermittent and arrhythmia is rarely captured unless an ECG is performed at the time of ongoing symptoms. Based on the frequency of symptoms, a 24-hour Holter monitor or a patient-activated event recorder for up to 2 weeks or longer may detect the event, yielding a diagnosis (16). Approximately, half of pregnant women with palpitations demonstrate premature atrial beats and nonsustained arrhythmias (3). Asymptomatic incidental arrhythmias should not be treated unless life threatening.

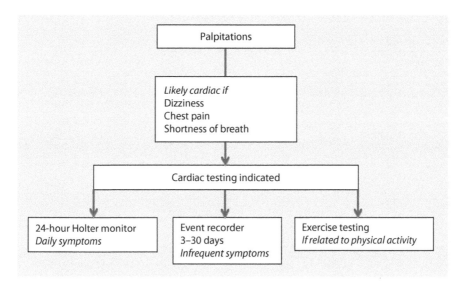

FIGURE 5.1    Approach to a patient with palpitations.

## Limitations of Physical Examination in Pregnancy

Pregnancy causes increase in heart rate, cardiac output, and plasma volume and reduced peripheral vascular resistance that leads to the mild dilation of the heart and changes in heart sounds. In the latter half of pregnancy, 90% of pregnant women have a systolic flow murmur, 80% have a third heart sound, and many will have a loud first heart sound with an exaggerated split (17,18). Pregnant women may have dependent edema, visible neck veins, and cardiomegaly. ECG often shows subtle changes, including leftward axis deviation due to the gravid uterus elevating the diaphragm and rotating the heart. The PR and QT intervals shorten with increased heart rate of pregnancy, and there may be nonspecific ST-segment and T-wave abnormalities (19). Differentiating normal pregnancy changes from an abnormal exam suggestive of cardiac disease may be challenging for the preceding reasons (Table 5.1). For general guidance, abnormal historical and exam findings may include severe dyspnea, exertion-related chest pain or syncope, paroxysmal nocturnal dyspnea, hemoptysis, cyanosis, clubbing, fourth heart sounds, diastolic murmurs, sustained cardiac arrhythmias, and loud, harsh systolic murmurs (20). Consultation with a cardiologist or an electrophysiologist is mandatory for accurate diagnosis and management of arrhythmias.

## Women with Structural Heart Disease

Arrhythmia is one of the five independent predictors of a cardiac event during pregnancy and should therefore be seriously approached (21). Overall, patients with a history of a structural heart defect have a 4.5% risk of an arrhythmia, with an approximately 15% risk for patients with surgically corrected hypoplastic left heart syndrome and transposition of the great vessels (4). Infection, hemorrhage, and pneumonia pose a great risk for life-threatening events in these patients due to the stress placed on an already strained cardiovascular system. To aid in identifying patients without a prior diagnosis and with genetic propensity for life-threatening arrhythmias, obtain a family history that concentrates on unexplained sudden premature deaths. Preconception counseling is of paramount importance for preexisting cardiac conditions and includes the evaluation and discussion of the risk and benefits of continuation versus discontinuation of antiarrhythmic medications.

TABLE 5.1

Normal Pregnancy Changes versus Those Suggestive of Cardiovascular Disease

| **Normal Pregnancy** | **Indicative of Cardiovascular Disease** |
|---|---|
| *Symptoms* | |
| Palpitations | Incapacitating palpitations |
| Fatigue | Progressive worsening; shortness of breath |
| Decreased exercise capacity | Paroxysmal nocturnal dyspnea |
| Light-headedness, near syncope | Chest pain with exertion |
| Shortness of breath | Syncope preceded by palpitations |
| Orthopnea | Hemoptysis |
| *Signs* | |
| Distended neck veins | Abnormal venous pulsations |
| Increased intensity of S1 | Loud systolic murmur |
| Exaggerated splitting of S2 | Any diastolic murmur |
| Mid-systolic murmur (lower left sternal border) | Ejection clicks; opening snap |
| Third heart sound | Sustained right or left ventricular heave |
| Palpable right ventricular impulse | Cyanosis or clubbing |
| *ECG* | |
| QRS axis deviation | Arrhythmia |
| Small Q and inverted P in lead III abolished by respiration | Heart blocks |
| Sinus tachycardia | |
| Arrhythmias | |
| *Echocardiography* | |
| Slight increase in systolic and diastolic left ventricular dimensions | Significantly dilated or hypertrophied heart |
| Moderate increase in sizes of right atrium, right ventricle, and left atrium | Significant valve abnormalities |
| Functional pulmonary, tricuspid and mitral regurgitation | |

## Management of Arrhythmias

There is a lack of randomized trials for treatment strategies in pregnant women and therefore most guidelines on observational studies, case reports, and clinical experience. In general, the approach to the treatment of arrhythmias is similar to that of nonpregnant women. Treatment decisions depend on the frequency, duration, and tolerability of the arrhythmia, including hemodynamic compromise.

## Antiarrhythmic Drugs

There are limited data on antiarrhythmic drugs in pregnancy, particularly in regard to the safety of the developing fetus. Organogenesis occurs in the first trimester, and during this time, the fetus is most sensitive to the effects of teratogens and drugs (22). The risk–benefit ratio of medications should be carefully analyzed based on the stage of pregnancy; often, physicians opt for older medications with longer safety records, at the lowest effective dose (Table 5.2; (23)).

## Direct-Current Cardioversion

Cardioversion is appropriate during any trimester of pregnancy primarily indicated for either drug-refractory arrhythmias or hemodynamically unstable tachyarrhythmia (24). Cardioversion does not compromise the blood flow to the fetus (25). In viable pregnancies, however, fetal monitoring is recommended due to a rare occurrence of fetal arrhythmia and the potential for uterine contractions (26,27).

**TABLE 5.2**

Commonly Used Antiarrhythmic Drugs and Their Safety in Pregnancy

| Drug | FDA Risk Category | Fetal Effects | Lactation |
|------|------|------|------|
| Adenosine | C | No reported effects | Limited data<br>Probably compatible due to short half-life |
| Beta-blockers | C, D | Fetal bradycardia, intrauterine growth restriction, low placental weight | Compatible with breastfeeding<br>May cause neonatal bradycardia |
| Digoxin | C | No reported effects | Compatible with breastfeeding |
| Verapamil | C | No reported effects | Compatible |
| Ibutilide | C | Limited data | No data |
| Flecainide | C | Limited data<br>Case reports of fetal SVT | Limited data<br>Probably compatible |
| Procainamide | C | No reported effects | Compatible with breastfeeding |
| Quinidine | C | Miscarriage, preterm labor, transient fetal thrombocytopenia, and damage to the eighth cranial nerve | Compatible with breastfeeding |
| Sotatol | B | Limited data<br>Case reports of fetal death, neurological morbidity, and newborn bradycardia | Compatible with breastfeeding |
| Amiodarone | D | Intrauterine growth restriction, fetal thyroid disorder, goiter, and prolonged QT in the newborn | Not compatible |

*Source:* US Food and Drug Administration classification of drug risk. From Office on Women's Health in the US Department of Health and Human Services, *Pregnancy and medicines fact sheet*, Available from: http://womenshealth.gov /publications/our-publications/fact-sheet/pregnancy-medicines.html.

## Pacemakers

Pacemakers can be safely placed throughout the pregnancy. Fetal risks due to radiation exposure are often a concern for providers and patients due to the general use of fluoroscopy during this procedure. Risks for miscarriage, fetal anomalies, and/or growth restriction are not increased until the total radiation exposure to the fetus exceeds 50 mGy or 5 rad (28). The pacemaker can also be placed with minimal radiation exposure. Abdominal shielding is often used to decrease the exposure to scattered radiation.

## Cardiac Ablation

There is reluctance to perform radio-frequency catheter ablation during pregnancy despite the high success rates outside of pregnancy for drug refractory or poorly tolerated supraventricular or VT. This procedure should be considered in these precarious situations (29). Radiation exposure has been found to be low, at less than 1 mGy (30). There have been recent technical innovations that minimize radiation exposure by using limited fluoroscopy, echocardiogram guidance, or nonfluoroscopic three-dimensional mapping systems (31–33). These advancements are decreasing the hesitation in performing ablations during pregnancy.

## Implantable Cardioverter Defibrillators

An implantable cardioverter defibrillator (ICD) is used to treat sustained or malignant ventricular arrhythmias to prevent sudden cardiac arrest. Patients with ICDs in place have good pregnancy outcomes without an increased risk of major ICD-related complications (34–36). The placement of an ICD is preferred prior to conception or during pregnancy if indicated. An external wearable device (life vest) can also be used awaiting the permanent placement of ICD or if arrhythmia is thought to be reversible or of short duration.

## Specific Arrhythmias

### Premature Atrial Contractions

Premature atrial contractions (PACs) are frequently encountered in pregnancy. In one study of pregnant women with symptoms versus those with isolated murmur, PACs were seen in 56% of pregnant women with symptoms and 58% of those with an isolated murmur during 24-hour Holter monitoring. The investigators found a significant reduction postpartum (3). Most women with PAC tend to be asymptomatic, and therapy is recommended only in the presence of intolerable symptoms. Cardioselective beta-blockers, such as metoprolol, can safely be used. Prior to initiating treatment, all potential precipitators such as caffeine, tobacco, or other stimulants must be discontinued (24) (Table 5.3).

### Supraventricular Tachycardia

SVT is the most common sustained arrhythmia encountered during pregnancy and is the most common arrhythmia in a structurally normal heart. The recurrence rate of symptomatic SVT has been found to be 22–50% with increased prevalence in patients with structural heart disease (37,38). The most common etiology is the presence of reentrant accessory pathway. The first step in the management of SVT is attempting vagal maneuvers followed by the standard doses of adenosine and, only if refractory to the initial maneuvers or if hemodynamically unstable, the use of direct-current cardioversion is recommended (39). Metoprolol, verapamil, digoxin, and ibutilide have also been used as the next-line acute agents, with data suggesting safety in pregnancy (13,40). In order to prevent frequent recurrent symptomatic episodes of SVT, atrioventricular-nodal blocking agents such as metoprolol or verapamil can be used (24).

### Atrial Fibrillation and Flutter

Atrial fibrillation and flutter are uncommon in pregnancy and are usually associated with a structural cardiac defect, i.e., congenital or valvular heart disease. Usually, the patient presents with tachycardia and/or pulmonary edema. More than 50% of patients with prior history of atrial fibrillation will have a symptomatic recurrence during pregnancy that warrants prompt evaluation. The most important complications include sustained symptomatic tachycardia and the risk of thromboembolism (41). Management includes the control of heart rate, the restoration of sinus rhythm, and the therapeutic levels of anticoagulation to prevent stroke or peripheral arterial embolization. A short duration of atrial fibrillation may respond to either electrical or pharmacological cardioversion. Medical therapy includes digoxin and a beta-blocker or nondihydropyridine calcium channel antagonist to control the rapid ventricular rate response (42,43). Thromboembolism prophylaxis is ensured with the use of anticoagulation agents or aspirin therapy based on the $CHA_2DS_2$-VASc score (Table 5.4) (43). In pregnancy, rhythm control is

TABLE 5.3

Arrhythmias in Pregnancy

| Arrhythmia | Frequency | Treatment | Prognosis |
|---|---|---|---|
| PACs | Most common in pregnancy; usually asymptomatic | Beta-blockers for symptom control | Excellent |
| SVT | Most common sustained arrhythmia | Vagal maneuvers; adenosine; cardioversion; beta-blockers; calcium channel blockers; ibutilide | Good |
| Atrial fibrillation and flutter | Uncommon; usually underlying structural cardiac defect | Beta-blockers; calcium channel blockers; digoxin; cardioversion; ibutilide; flecainide | Good |
| VT | Rare; usually underlying structural cardiac defect | Beta-blockers; cardioversion; amiodarone; ICD | Fair |
| Bradycardia and heart blocks | Rare | Pacemaker for symptoms | Good |

TABLE 5.4

Risk Assessment for Stroke in Non-Valvular Atrial Fibrillation

| $CHA_2DS_2$-VASc | Score |
|---|---|
| Congestive heart failure | 1 |
| Hypertension | 1 |
| Age > 75 years (not applicable to obstetrical population) | 2 |
| Diabetes | 1 |
| Stroke/transient ischemic attack/thromboembolic | 2 |
| Vascular disease (myocardial infarction, peripheral arterial disease, aortic plaque) | 1 |
| Age 65–74 years (not applicable to obstetrical population) | 1 |
| Sex category (female) | 1 |

obtained with the use of ibutilide, class 1A (quinidine, procainamide) or 1C (flecainide, propafenone), to block the reentry conduction pathways that are usually the cause of tachycardia in this setting (42).

## Ventricular Tachycardia

VT generally occurs in a setting of structural heart defect and therefore tends to recur particularly if diagnosed prior to pregnancy. The risk of recurrent VT is nearly 30% during pregnancy (37). Cardioversion is preferred in hemodynamically unstable patients. Stable patients are managed with medications such as beta-blockers, procainamide, and flecainide. Sustained ventricular arrhythmias may lead to cardiac arrest. Due to the high risk for sudden cardiac death, patients with sustained VT are candidates for external defibrillator or the placement of an ICD. These devices can be placed with minimal radiation, and the information known on ICDs during pregnancy is overall reassuring (35,44).

## Bradycardia

Defined as a heart rate less than 60, sinus bradycardia is an uncommon problem during pregnancy. It may however occur during labor and may persist for several days postpartum (41). Bradycardia is typically asymptomatic and does not generally require intervention. Symptomatic bradycardia needs prompt treatment according to advanced cardiac life support guidelines (45). Transcutaneous and transvenous pacemakers are considered safe and should be used when appropriate. In a setting of complete heart block, the heart rate is generally less than 50 and is symptomatic; a pacemaker insertion is warranted (46,47).

## Conduction Disorders

There is no association between first- and second-degree atrioventricular block or complete heart block and pregnancy. Second-degree Mobitz type 1 (Wenckebach) is more commonly seen and is usually considered benign. It rarely progresses to complete heart block and is therefore conservatively managed. Mobitz type 2 is uncommon but can progress to complete heart block, and, therefore, a permanent pacemaker is often recommended even in asymptomatic patients. Complete heart block is rarely diagnosed for the first time in pregnancy and is usually associated with prior cardiac surgery, CHD, myocardial infarction, cardiomyopathy, drugs, metabolic imbalance, and acute infection (48). However, 30% of cases remain undetectable until adulthood (49). In pregnancy, pacemakers are usually recommended for symptoms or in the presence of slow, wide complex escape rhythm (50).

## Cardiac Arrest

We recommend following the 2015 American Heart Association's guidelines in pregnancy (45). In general, salient principles include quicker maternal deoxygenation in pregnancy, maneuvers to relieve aortocaval uterine compression, and performing a perimortem cesarean delivery for maternal benefit at 4 minutes into the arrest when the estimated gestational age of the fetus is greater than 20 weeks.

## In Summary

The incidence of cardiac arrhythmias is higher during pregnancy and highest in pregnant women with a history of heart disease. Arrhythmia and the common symptoms accompanying arrhythmia, such as palpitations, chest pain, and shortness of breath, pose a challenge to obstetric care providers as normal symptoms of pregnancy overlap with these complaints. Fortunately, most arrhythmias during pregnancy are benign and do not require therapy. Patients should be thoroughly evaluated based on the frequency and severity of symptoms, cardiac disease risk factors, and physical examination findings. There are increasing data on the safety of most medications and device therapy in pregnancy. In general, arrhythmias can be safely managed in a multidisciplinary manner with input from maternal–fetal medicine, anesthesia, and cardiology.

## REFERENCES

1. Al-Yaseen E, Al-Na'ar A, Hassan M, Al-Ostad G, Ibrahim E. Palpitation in pregnancy: Experience in one major hospital in Kuwait. *Med J Islam Repub Iran*. 2013; 27(1):31-34.
2. Choi HS, Han SS, Choi HA, Kim HS, Lee CG, Kim YY et al. Dyspnea and palpitation during pregnancy. *Korean J Intern Med*. 2001; 16(4):247-249.
3. Shotan A, Ostrzega E, Mehra A, Johnson JV, Elkayam U. Incidence of arrhythmias in normal pregnancy and relation to palpitations, dizziness, and syncope. *Am J Cardiol*. 1997; 79(8):1061-1064.
4. Drenthen W, Boersma E, Balci A, Moons P, Roos-Hesselink JW, Mulder BJ et al. Predictors of pregnancy complications in women with congenital heart disease. *Eur Heart J*. 2010; 31(17): 2124-2132.
5. Drenthen W, Pieper PG, Roos-Hesselink JW, van Lottum WA, Voors AA, Mulder BJ et al. Outcome of pregnancy in women with congenital heart disease: A literature review. *J Am Coll Cardiol*. 2007; 49(24):2303-2311.
6. Siu SC, Sermer M, Colman JM, Alvarez AN, Mercier LA, Morton BC et al. Prospective multicenter study of pregnancy outcomes in women with heart disease. *Circulation*. 2001; 104(5):515-521.
7. Sanghavi M, Rutherford JD. Cardiovascular physiology of pregnancy. *Circulation*. 2014; 130(12): 1003-1008.
8. Mahendru AA, Everett TR, Wilkinson IB, Lees CC, McEniery CM. A longitudinal study of maternal cardiovascular function from preconception to the postpartum period. *J Hypertens*. 2014; 32(4):849-856.
9. Turner AS, Watson OF, Adey HS, Cottle LP, Spence R. The prevalence of disturbance of cardiac rhythm in randomly selected New Zealand adults. *N Z Med J*. 1981; 93(682):253-255.
10. Kroenke K, Arrington ME, Mangelsdorff AD. The prevalence of symptoms in medical outpatients and the adequacy of therapy. *Arch Intern Med*. 1990; 150(8):1685-1689.
11. Li JM, Nguyen C, Joglar JA, Hamdan MH, Page RL. Frequency and outcome of arrhythmias complicating admission during pregnancy: Experience from a high-volume and ethnically-diverse obstetric service. *Clin Cardiol*. 2008; 31(11):538-541.
12. Gowda RM, Khan IA, Mehta NJ, Vasavada BC, Sacchi TJ. Cardiac arrhythmias in pregnancy: Clinical and therapeutic considerations. *Int J Cardiol*. 2003; 88(2-3):129-133.
13. Knotts RJ, Garan H. Cardiac arrhythmias in pregnancy. *Semin Perinatol*. 2014; 38(5):285-288.
14. Weber BE, Kapoor WN. Evaluation and outcomes of patients with palpitations. *Am J Med*. 1996; 100(2):138-148.
15. Mayou R, Sprigings D, Birkhead J, Price J. Characteristics of patients presenting to a cardiac clinic with palpitation. *QJM*. 2003; 96(2):115-123.
16. Zimetbaum PJ, Kim KY, Josephson ME, Goldberger AL, Cohen DJ. Diagnostic yield and optimal duration of continuous-loop event monitoring for the diagnosis of palpitations: A cost-effectiveness analysis. *Ann Intern Med*. 1998; 128(11):890-895.
17. Nishimura RA, Otto CM, Bonow RO, Carabello BA, Erwin JP III, Guyton RA et al. 2014 AHA/ACC guideline for the management of patients with valvular heart disease: A report of the American College of Cardiology/American Heart Association Task Force on Practice Guidelines. *J Thorac Cardiovasc Surg*. 2014; 148(1):e1-e132.
18. Cutforth R, MacDonald CB. Heart sounds and murmurs in pregnancy. *Am Heart J*. 1966; 71(6):741-747.

19. Carruth JE, Mivis SB, Brogan DR, Wenger NK. The electrocardiogram in normal pregnancy. *Am Heart J.* 1981; 102(6 Pt 1):1075-1078.
20. Thorne SA. Pregnancy in heart disease. *Heart.* 2004; 90(4):450-456.
21. Siu SC, Sermer M, Harrison DA, Grigoriadis E, Liu G, Sorensen S et al. Risk and predictors for pregnancy-related complications in women with heart disease. *Circulation.* 1997; 96(9):2789-2794.
22. Joglar JA, Page RL. Treatment of cardiac arrhythmias during pregnancy: Safety considerations. *Drug Saf.* 1999; 20(1):85-94.
23. Office on Women's Health in the US Department of Health and Human Services. *Pregnancy and medicines fact sheet.* Available from: http://womenshealth.gov/publications/our-publications/fact-sheet/pregnancy-medicines.html.
24. Cox JL, Gardner MJ. Treatment of cardiac arrhythmias during pregnancy. *Prog Cardiovasc Dis.* 1993; 36(2):137-178.
25. Wang YC, Chen CH, Su HY, Yu MH. The impact of maternal cardioversion on fetal haemodynamics. *Eur J Obstet Gynecol Reprod Biol.* 2006; 126(2):268-269.
26. Page RL. Treatment of arrhythmias during pregnancy. *Am Heart J.* 1995; 130(4):871-876.
27. Barnes EJ, Eben F, Patterson D. Direct current cardioversion during pregnancy should be performed with facilities available for fetal monitoring and emergency caesarean section. *BJOG.* 2002; 109(12):1406-1407.
28. ACOG Committee on Obstetric Practice. ACOG Committee Opinion. Number 299, September 2004 (replaces No. 158, September 1995): Guidelines for diagnostic imaging during pregnancy. *Obstet Gynecol.* 2004; 104(3):647-651.
29. Driver K, Chisholm CA, Darby AE, Malhotra R, Dimarco JP, Ferguson JD. Catheter ablation of arrhythmia during pregnancy. *J Cardiovasc Electrophysiol.* 2015; 26(6):698-702.
30. Damilakis J, Theocharopoulos N, Perisinakis K, Manios E, Dimitriou P, Vardas P et al. Conceptus radiation dose and risk from cardiac catheter ablation procedures. *Circulation.* 2001; 104(8):893-897.
31. Casella M, Dello Russo A, Pelargonio G, Del Greco M, Zingarini G, Piacenti M et al. Near zero fluoroscopic exposure during catheter ablation of supraventricular arrhythmias: The no-party multicentre randomized trial. *Europace.* 2016; 18(10):1565-1572.
32. Bigelow AM, Crane SS, Khoury FR, Clark JM. Catheter ablation of supraventricular tachycardia without fluoroscopy during pregnancy. *Obstet Gynecol.* 2015; 125(6):1338-1341.
33. Raman AS, Sharma S, Hariharan R. Minimal use of fluoroscopy to reduce fetal radiation exposure during radiofrequency catheter ablation of maternal supraventricular tachycardia. *Tex Heart Inst J.* 2015; 42(2):152-154.
34. Miyoshi T, Kamiya CA, Katsuragi S, Ueda H, Kobayashi Y, Horiuchi C et al. Safety and efficacy of implantable cardioverter-defibrillator during pregnancy and after delivery. *Circ J.* 2013; 77(5):1166-1170.
35. Natale A, Davidson T, Geiger MJ, Newby K. Implantable cardioverter-defibrillators and pregnancy: A safe combination? *Circulation.* 1997; 96(9):2808-2812.
36. Piper JM, Berkus M, Ridgway LE III. Pregnancy complicated by chronic cardiomyopathy and an automatic implantable cardioverter defibrillator. *Am J Obstet Gynecol.* 1992; 167(2):506-507.
37. Silversides CK, Harris L, Haberer K, Sermer M, Colman JM, Siu SC. Recurrence rates of arrhythmias during pregnancy in women with previous tachyarrhythmia and impact on fetal and neonatal outcomes. *Am J Cardiol.* 2006; 97(8):1206-1212.
38. Lee SH, Chen SA, Wu TJ, Chiang CE, Cheng CC, Tai CT et al. Effects of pregnancy on first onset and symptoms of paroxysmal supraventricular tachycardia. *Am J Cardiol.* 1995; 76(10):675-678.
39. Page RL, Joglar JA, Caldwell MA, Calkins H, Conti JB, Deal BJ et al. 2015 ACC/AHA/HRS Guideline for the management of adult patients with supraventricular tachycardia: A report of the American College of Cardiology/American Heart Association Task Force on Clinical Practice Guidelines and the Heart Rhythm Society. *J Am Coll Cardiol.* 2016; 67(13):e27-e115.
40. Kockova R, Kocka V, Kiernan T, Fahy GJ. Ibutilide-induced cardioversion of atrial fibrillation during pregnancy. *J Cardiovasc Electrophysiol.* 2007; 18(5):545-547.
41. Mendelson CL. Disorders of the heartbeat during pregnancy. *Am J Obstet Gynecol.* 1956; 72(6):1268-1301.
42. European Society of Gynecology, Association for European Paediatric Cardiology, German Society for Gender Medicine, Regitz-Zagrosek V, Blomstrom Lundqvist C, Borghi C et al. ESC Guidelines on the management of cardiovascular diseases during pregnancy: The Task Force on the Management of Cardiovascular Diseases during Pregnancy of the European Society of Cardiology (ESC). *Eur Heart J.* 2011; 32(24):3147-3197.

43. Fuster V, Ryden LE, Cannom DS, Crijns HJ, Curtis AB, Ellenbogen KA et al. ACC/AHA/ESC 2006 guidelines for the management of patients with atrial fibrillation: A report of the American College of Cardiology/American Heart Association Task Force on Practice Guidelines and the European Society of Cardiology Committee for Practice Guidelines (Writing Committee to Revise the 2001 Guidelines for the Management of Patients with Atrial Fibrillation). *Europace.* 2006; 8(9):651-745.

44. Abello M, Peinado R, Merino JL, Gnoatto M, Mateos M, Silvestre J et al. Cardioverter defibrillator implantation in a pregnant woman guided with transesophageal echocardiography. *Pacing Clin Electrophysiol.* 2003; 26(9):1913-1914.

45. Jeejeebhoy FM, Zelop CM, Lipman S, Carvalho B, Joglar J, Mhyre JM et al. Cardiac arrest in pregnancy: A scientific statement from the American Heart Association. *Circulation.* 2015; 132(18):1747-1773.

46. Antonelli D, Bloch L, Rosenfeld T. Implantation of permanent dual chamber pacemaker in a pregnant woman by transesophageal echocardiographic guidance. *Pacing Clin Electrophysiol.* 1999; 22(3):534-535.

47. Schroeder JS, Harrison DC. Repeated cardioversion during pregnancy: Treatment of refractory paroxysmal atrial tachycardia during 3 successive pregnancies. *Am J Cardiol.* 1971; 27(4):445-446.

48. Eddy WA, Frankenfeld RH. Congenital complete heart block in pregnancy. *Am J Obstet Gynecol.* 1977; 128(2):223-225.

49. Michaelsson M, Jonzon A, Riesenfeld T. Isolated congenital complete atrioventricular block in adult life: A prospective study. *Circulation.* 1995; 92(3):442-449.

50. Jaffe R, Gruber A, Fejgin M, Altaras M, Ben-Aderet N. Pregnancy with an artificial pacemaker. *Obstet Gynecol Surv.* 1987; 42(3):137-139.

# 6

## Chest Pain

**Afshan B. Hameed, MD, FACC, FACOG**

CONTENTS

## Introduction

Cardiovascular disease complicates about 1–4% of pregnancies and is the leading cause of pregnancy-related deaths in the United States (1,2). Chest pain is not only the most common symptom of heart disease but also the most frequent cause of emergency department (ED) visits (3). The evaluation of chest pain is challenging as the etiology may range from benign heart burn, which is a common complaint in pregnancy, to a life-threatening condition such as acute coronary syndrome (ACS) or aortic dissection. The purpose of this chapter is to provide a systematic approach to addressing this relatively common complaint in pregnancy.

## Cardiovascular Physiology of Pregnancy

An understanding of the physiological changes in pregnancy is of utmost importance to manage a pregnant woman with non-pregnancy-related complaints. Cardiovascular changes during pregnancy include an increase in heart rate, stroke volume, and cardiac output along with a decrease in systemic vascular resistance, systemic blood pressure, and blood volume expansion (4). Pregnancy is also a hypercoagulable state with 4- to 10-fold increased risk of a thromboembolic event (5). These evolutionary changes provide more blood flow to the placenta/fetus and at the same time prevents excessive blood loss at the time of delivery.

## Evaluation of Chest Pain in Pregnancy

Chest pain is a common complaint in pregnancy. The spectrum of chest pain varies from benign causes such as gastroesophageal reflux disease (GERD) to the life-threatening diagnosis of acute myocardial infarction (MI) (Table 6.1). Fortunately, the most common etiology of chest pain in pregnancy is GERD, aggravated by the progesterone-mediated relaxation of lowering the lower esophageal sphincter tone.

TABLE 6.1

Differential Diagnosis of Chest Pain during Pregnancy

| Cardiac | ACS[a] |
|---|---|
| | Pericarditis |
| | Myocarditis |
| Vascular | Dissection (coronary, aortic)[a] |
| | PE[a] |
| | Pulmonary hypertension |
| Pulmonary | Pneumonia |
| | Pleurisy |
| | Pneumothorax |
| | Tumor |
| Musculoskeletal | Costochondritis, spine or shoulder arthritis |
| Gastrointestinal | Reflux, peptic ulcer, esophageal spasm, Mallory–Weiss tear, pancreatitis, biliary colic |
| Miscellaneous | Breast, herpes zoster |

[a]  Life-threatening acute diagnosis requiring immediate recognition and treatment.

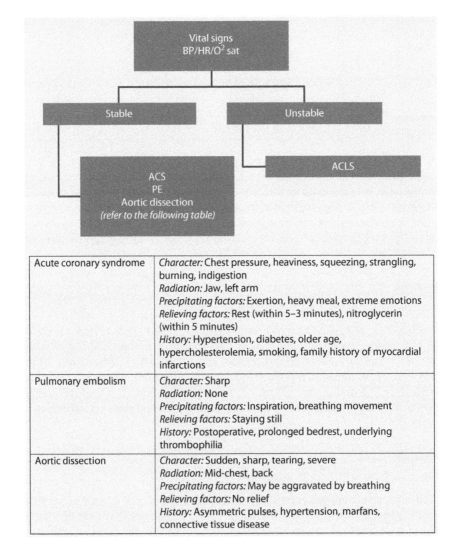

FIGURE 6.1   Chest pain algorithm.

The challenge for the healthcare provider evaluating pregnant and postpartum women with chest pain is to keep these physiological changes in mind while ruling out the few life-threatening causes of chest pain such as ACS (the term that encompasses the disease process that reduces blood flow to the heart including MI), pulmonary embolism (PE), and aortic dissection.

Chest pain should follow the same general principles as considered in the nonpregnant population (Figure 6.1). A thorough medical history should be obtained, focusing on the risk factors for cardiac disease such as age, cardiac history, family history, smoking, and diabetes. Vital signs should be evaluated. Physical examination including the auscultation of the heart, neck, and lungs and evaluating for peripheral edema provides valuable information including extra heart sounds or evidence of heart failure. Coexisting medical complications should be used in risk assessment. The vast majority of investigations and treatments should not be withheld in pregnancy, including diagnostics that involve radiation. Women with medical problems in pregnancy should be managed with a multidisciplinary team approach.

The following features are useful in the evaluation of chest pain:

1. Type of chest pain: Burning, pressure, heaviness, sharp, dull ache, or tearing
2. Location of chest pain: Upper epigastric, lower, left or right chest, or back
3. Radiation: To the left arm or to the jaw or to the back
4. Associated symptoms: Nausea, vomiting, diaphoresis, palpitations, shortness of breath, dizziness or syncope
5. Aggravating or relieving factors: Emotion, exercise, breathing, lying down, or standing up
6. Duration of chest pain: All day, all night, instantaneous, prolonged, minutes or hours

The differential diagnosis of chest pain is outlined in Table 6.2. The goal for the healthcare provider is to identify these three most important and deadly causes of chest pain, i.e., myocardial ischemia/infarction (coronary artery dissection, atherosclerosis less common), aortic dissection (Marfans syndrome, collagen vascular diseases, pregnancy), and PE to avoid a catastrophic event.

Pregnant women may present with a nonclassic presentation of ACS. These symptoms may include chest pain lasting from seconds to over 12 hours, worsening with positional change or may describe it as "sharp or stabbing." Associated symptoms of gastrointestinal complaints; nonspecific fatigue or dizziness; and jaw, neck, or back pain were more common in women with ACSs (6). A study in the United Kingdom found that a significant number of pregnant women with ACS symptoms were not assessed with an electrocardiogram (ECG) or cardiac biomarkers, and half of those who died had received substandard care for cardiac symptoms (7).

The ECG in normal pregnancy may show nonspecific T-wave inversions, axis deviation, or other changes due to an elevated diaphragm or chamber dilation, making the diagnosis of ischemia challenging (8). Indications for additional diagnostic testing include a history of cardiac disease, symptoms excessive from the norm, pathological murmur, evidence of heart failure on exam, and oxygen desaturation in the absence of pulmonary disease. Laboratory testing should include a complete blood count to evaluate for anemia, a metabolic panel in the setting of hypertension to evaluate for HELLP (hemolysis, elevated liver enzymes, and low platelet count)/acute fatty liver as these may present with acute severe epigastric/lower chest pain. Additionally, arterial blood gas (ABG), chest X-ray, or pulmonary function tests may be considered if pulmonary disease is suspected.

Administering medications for acid reflux such as calcium carbonate or oral viscous lidocaine may be helpful in assisting to tease out a gastrointestinal cause. ECGs are usually nonspecific but may detect the evidence of right heart strain related to PE and ST segment changes due to myocardial ischemia or an arrhythmia. Continuous ECG monitoring may be indicated in the event that a cardiac arrhythmia is suspected.

## Acute Myocardial Infarction

The risk of MI increases by threefold during pregnancy and postpartum period with an incidence of 1:16,000 of all deliveries (9,10). Risk factors in pregnancy-related MI include age of >30 years,

TABLE 6.2

Diagnostic Tests for Acute Chest Pain

| | |
|---|---|
| ACS | ECG |
| | Troponin levels |
| | ±Coronary angiogram |
| |   Percutaneous coronary intervention[a] |
| |   Coronary artery by-pass graft |
| PE | ECG |
| | ABG |
| | CT angiogram |
| | V/Q scan |
| | Lower extremity duplex |
| | D-dimer[b] |
| Aortic dissection | ECG |
| | Transesophageal echocardiogram |
| | MR angiogram |
| | CT angiogram |

[a] Selected cases with ongoing symptoms after multidisciplinary consultation with cardiology, cardiothoracic surgery, anesthesia, maternal–fetal medicine, and neonatology.

[b] D-dimer may be useful if within normal limits in pregnancy.

hyperlipidemia, hypertension, preeclampsia, diabetes, and obesity. In pregnant women with MI, the most common etiology is coronary dissection (43%) followed by atherosclerosis in 27% patients (11–14). This is in contrast to the atherosclerosis as the predominant cause outside of pregnancy. The propensity for coronary artery dissection is thought to be mediated through the hormone-induced changes in the connective tissue of the coronary arteries. The vast majority in pregnancy presents as ST segment elevation MI and high prevalence of heart failure, arrhythmias, and cardiogenic shock (11,15).

Acute MI most frequently occurs during the third trimester and within 6 weeks postpartum (16). The diagnosis of an MI is often delayed in pregnancy due to low suspicion on account of rarity and attributing cardiovascular symptoms to normal pregnancy changes. Diagnosis should be guided by the same principles as used for the general population by identifying ischemic symptoms, electrocardiographic abnormalities, and elevations in cardiac biomarkers (15). It should be kept in mind that creatine kinase myocardial B fraction (MB) isoenzyme is normally increased in the immediate postpartum period, peaking at 24 hours postpartum. Troponin levels, on the other hand, remain within the normal range during pregnancy and postpartum period, and therefore, any elevations in the troponin levels should be further evaluated (17,18). If the ECG or biomarkers are nondiagnostic, a stress test or an echocardiogram may be used to evaluate for ischemia-related wall motion abnormalities. In women with recent or suspected MI, care should be carefully coordinated with cardiology, emergency, and obstetric teams.

The management of MI in pregnancy is similar to that of the general population with a focus on reperfusion with either medications, percutaneous coronary intervention, or coronary artery bypass surgery (10,19,20). Management should proceed with caution due to the known fragility of the coronary blood vessels in pregnancy with a tendency for coronary dissection (11). Thrombolytic therapy is relatively contraindicated in pregnancy due to the risk of abruption, fetal loss, and bleeding complications.

Medications commonly used in the management of MIs may safely be used in pregnancy including aspirin, beta-blockers, anticoagulation, nitrates, and morphine. Thrombolytic therapy, while used, is relatively contraindicated due to the slight increased risk of maternal bleeding, preterm delivery, or fetal loss. Angiotensin-converting enzyme inhibitors, angiotensin II receptor blockers, and statins are contraindicated in pregnancy. Medications that cause coronary vasoconstriction such as methergine and prostaglandin should be avoided.

There is an increased risk of maternal death if delivery occurs within 2 weeks of an infarction, and therefore, elective delivery should not be performed. The fetus should be monitored if at a viable gestational age. There should be a delivery plan in place for the event of maternal or fetal deterioration. At the time of delivery, the goals are minimization of the cardiac workload, which is accomplished by supplemental oxygen, avoiding the supine position but in the left lateral position, and medical management of hypertension. It is best to avoid tachycardia, epidural anesthesia, and instrumented vaginal delivery, and only in unstable cases is a cesarean section indicated (9).

## Pulmonary Embolism

Thromboembolism encompasses deep venous thrombosis and PE, with a prevalence of 0.5–2.0 per 1000 pregnancies, and accounts for 9% of maternal deaths in the United States (21). Risk factors for venous thromboembolism (VTE) include personal history of thrombosis, thrombophilia, obesity, hypertension, smoking, operative delivery, and the physiological changes of pregnancy and postpartum period. Prior history of VTE and thrombophilia confers the highest risk for VTE in pregnancy (22,23).

Symptoms include chest pain, tachypnea, and tachycardia. ABG shows hypoxia with a wide A–a gradient in 80% of cases of PE. ECG may show nonspecific changes in 80%, and the classic S1Q3T3 is seen in only 15%.

Computed tomography (CT) angiography and ventilation–perfusion (V/Q) scan are the most commonly used initial tests for the diagnosis of PE in pregnancy with low radiation exposure to the fetus. Pulmonary angiogram remains the gold standard for diagnosing PE; however, utility is limited in pregnancy due to its invasive nature. Magnetic resonance angiogram may also be considered in some cases. Chest X-ray finding include infiltrate, effusion, or atelectasis. Occasionally, pleural-based wedge-shaped defect may be seen abutting the diaphragm in cases of lung infarction (Hampton's hump) or oligemia downstream from the embolus (Westermark's sign).

The diagnostic workup and treatment should proceed similar to that in nonpregnant individuals (Figure 6.2). If the clinical suspicion is high, pregnant woman should receive therapeutic anticoagulation

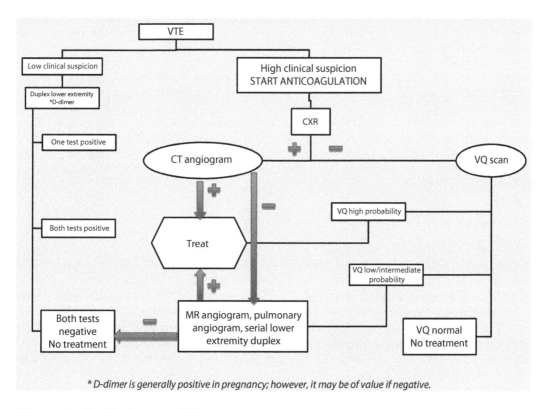

*\* D-dimer is generally positive in pregnancy; however, it may be of value if negative.*

FIGURE 6.2   Algorithm for suspected PE.

prior to/or while waiting for diagnostic testing. Further continuation, strength, and duration of anticoagulation are determined by a combination of the confirmation of the diagnosis of VTE and the underlying risk factors (21).

Anticoagulation options during pregnancy include unfractionated heparin, low-molecular weight heparin, and warfarin. Heparins are the preferred choice in pregnancy as these agents do not cross the placental barrier (24).

## Aortic Dissection

Aortic dissection is a rare life-threatening condition in pregnancy that may lead to mortality if not identified and managed in a timely manner. There are two types of aortic dissection based on the Stanford classification: Stanford type A involves the ascending aorta, and type B is distal to the left subclavian artery origin. The incidence of type A aortic dissection is 0.4 per 100,000 person years in pregnancy (25). If untreated, the mortality rate of proximal aortic dissection at the time of presentation is 15%, which may increase to 25% in the first 24 hours (26).

### Risk Factors

Although most cases of aortic dissection are related to an underlying connective tissue disorder, mainly Marfan's syndrome (27,28), it may complicate an otherwise normal healthy pregnancy (29). Other risk factors for aortic dissection include pregnancy, bicuspid aortic valve, connective tissue disorders, syncope, hypertension, trauma, and a family history of aneurysm (30). Aortic dissection is most commonly encountered in the third trimester of pregnancy and is thought to be due to the hormonal changes in the vessel wall in combination with the hemodynamic stress (31).

Aortic dissection typically presents as a severe, sharp, tearing chest pain, light-headedness, and/or syncope primarily due to pericardial tamponade (32).

Chest radiograph may not demonstrate a widened mediastinum, and transesophageal echocardiography is considered the gold standard for diagnosing aortic dissection (33). Other tests include magnetic resonance (MR) angiogram or a CT scan.

Rapid diagnosis and early intervention is the key to successful treatment and prevention of significant maternal morbidity and even mortality (34,35). A multidisciplinary team is essential to optimize both maternal and fetal outcomes. Immediate delivery may be indicated in selected cases (36). One acceptable approach is to proceed with indicated aortic repair without cesarean delivery prior to 28 weeks and to consider concomitant cesarean delivery after 32 weeks. Most cases require individual planning based on individual risk factors in a multidisciplinary setting. Type A aortic dissection involves the ascending aorta and may be associated with aortic valve insufficiency, and impaired coronary perfusions (37,38) are surgically managed. Type B aortic dissections are usually medically managed and are amenable to endovascular repair (38–40).

## Conclusions

Chest pain is a common complaint in pregnancy and one of the most frequent presenting symptoms in the ED. The spectrum of chest pain varies from benign causes such as GERD to the life-threatening diagnosis of aortic/coronary dissection in pregnancy. Fortunately, GERD is the most common etiology of chest pain in pregnancy; however, other diagnoses must be considered in the differential, and GERD should be a diagnosis of exclusion based on the features of chest pain. The challenge for the healthcare provider evaluating pregnant and postpartum women with chest pain is to keep the life-threatening conditions in mind along with the physiological changes that may impact the presenting symptoms and the diagnostic tests. A pregnant woman must be managed in a manner similar to the nonpregnant counterparts presenting with complaints of chest pain to the ED to prevent catastrophic consequences.

# REFERENCES

1. Creanga AA, Berg CJ, Syverson C, Seed K, Bruce FC, Callaghan WM. Pregnancy-related mortality in the United States, 2006–2010. *Obstet Gynecol.* 2015; 125(1):5-12.
2. Berg CJ, Callaghan WM, Syverson C, Henderson Z. Pregnancy-related mortality in the United States, 1998 to 2005. *Obstet Gynecol.* 2010; 116(6):1302-1309.
3. Bhuiya FA, Pitts SR, McCaig LF. Emergency department visits for chest pain and abdominal pain: United States, 1999–2008. *NCHS Data Brief.* 2010(43):1-8.
4. Sanghavi M, Rutherford JD. Cardiovascular physiology of pregnancy. *Circulation.* 2014; 130(12): 1003-1008.
5. Brenner B. Haemostatic changes in pregnancy. *Thromb Res.* 2004; 114(5–6):409-414.
6. Arslanian-Engoren C, Patel A, Fang J, Armstrong D, Kline-Rogers E, Duvernoy CS et al. Symptoms of men and women presenting with acute coronary syndromes. *Am J Cardiol.* 2006; 98(9):1177-1181.
7. Cantwell R, Clutton-Brock T, Cooper G, Dawson A, Drife J, Garrod D et al. Saving mothers' lives: Reviewing maternal deaths to make motherhood safer: 2006–2008: The Eighth Report of the Confidential Enquiries into Maternal Deaths in the United Kingdom. *BJOG.* 2011; 118(Suppl 1):1-203.
8. Sahni G. Chest pain syndromes in pregnancy. *Cardiol Clin.* 2012; 30(3):343-367.
9. Roth A, Elkayam U. Acute myocardial infarction associated with pregnancy. *J Am Coll Cardiol.* 2008; 52(3):171-180.
10. James AH, Jamison MG, Biswas MS, Brancazio LR, Swamy GK, Myers ER. Acute myocardial infarction in pregnancy: A United States population-based study. *Circulation.* 2006; 113(12):1564-1571.
11. Elkayam U, Jalnapurkar S, Barakkat MN, Khatri N, Kealey AJ, Mehra A et al. Pregnancy-associated acute myocardial infarction: A review of contemporary experience in 150 cases between 2006 and 2011. *Circulation.* 2014; 129(16):1695-1702.
12. Schmutz A, Quaas P, Grundmann S. Chest pain at 32 weeks' gestation: Pregnancy-related spontaneous coronary artery dissection. *Anaesthesist.* 2016; 65(9):690-695.
13. Magarkar V, Lathi P. A case of spontaneous coronary artery dissection in early pregnancy managed by PCI. *Indian Heart J.* 2016; 68 Suppl 2:S25-S27.
14. Regitz-Zagrosek V, Jaguszewska K, Preis K. Pregnancy-related spontaneous coronary artery dissection. *Eur Heart J.* 2015; 36(34):2273-2274.
15. Mihaljevic S, Radivojevic RC, Mihaljevic L. Acute coronary syndrome with ST-segment elevation in pregnancy: Anesthetic management of delivery. *Coll Antropol.* 2015; 39(2):447-450.
16. Ladner HE, Danielsen B, Gilbert WM. Acute myocardial infarction in pregnancy and the puerperium: A population-based study. *Obstet Gynecol.* 2005; 105(3):480-484.
17. Khan DA, Sharif MS, Khan FA. Diagnostic performance of high-sensitivity troponin T, myeloperoxidase, and pregnancy-associated plasma protein A assays for triage of patients with acute myocardial infarction. *Korean J Lab Med.* 2011; 31(3):172-178.
18. Shade GH, Jr., Ross G, Bever FN, Uddin Z, Devireddy L, Gardin JM. Troponin I in the diagnosis of acute myocardial infarction in pregnancy, labor, and post partum. *Am J Obstet Gynecol.* 2002; 187(6):1719-1720.
19. Chaithiraphan V, Gowda RM, Khan IA, Reimers CD. Peripartum acute myocardial infarction: Management perspective. *Am J Ther.* 2003; 10(1):75-77.
20. Sanchez-Ramos L, Chami YG, Bass TA, DelValle GO, Adair CD. Myocardial infarction during pregnancy: Management with transluminal coronary angioplasty and metallic intracoronary stents. *Am J Obstet Gynecol.* 1994; 171(5):1392-1393.
21. James A, Committee on Practice Bulletins—Obstetrics. Practice Bulletin No. 123: Thromboembolism in pregnancy. *Obstet Gynecol.* 2011; 118(3):718-729.
22. Pabinger I, Grafenhofer H, Kyrle PA, Quehenberger P, Mannhalter C, Lechner K et al. Temporary increase in the risk for recurrence during pregnancy in women with a history of venous thromboembolism. *Blood.* 2002; 100(3):1060-1062.
23. James AH. Thromboembolism in pregnancy: Recurrence risks, prevention and management. *Curr Opin Obstet Gynecol.* 2008; 20(6):550-556.
24. Greer IA. Venous thromboembolism and anticoagulant therapy in pregnancy. *Gend Med.* 2005; 2(Suppl A):S10-S17.
25. Thalmann M, Sodeck GH, Domanovits H, Grassberger M, Loewe C, Grimm M et al. Acute type A aortic dissection and pregnancy: A population-based study. *Eur J Cardiothorac Surg.* 2011; 39(6):e159-e163.

26. Pitt MP, Bonser RS. The natural history of thoracic aortic aneurysm disease: An overview. *J Card Surg.* 1997; 12(2 Suppl):270-278.

27. Immer FF, Bansi AG, Immer-Bansi AS, McDougall J, Zehr KJ, Schaff HV et al. Aortic dissection in pregnancy: Analysis of risk factors and outcome. *Ann Thorac Surg.* 2003; 76(1):309-314.

28. Kim SW, Kim D, Hong JM. Acute aortic dissection in pregnancy with the Marfan syndrome. *Korean J Thorac Cardiovasc Surg.* 2014; 47(3):291-293.

29. Kinney-Ham L, Nguyen HB, Steele R, Walters EL. Acute aortic dissection in third trimester pregnancy without risk factors. *West J Emerg Med.* 2011; 12(4):571-574.

30. Kamel H, Roman MJ, Pitcher A, Devereux RB. Pregnancy and the risk of aortic dissection or rupture: A cohort-crossover analysis. *Circulation.* 2016; 134(7):527-533.

31. Anderson RA, Fineron PW. Aortic dissection in pregnancy: Importance of pregnancy-induced changes in the vessel wall and bicuspid aortic valve in pathogenesis. *Br J Obstet Gynaecol.* 1994; 101(12):1085-1088.

32. Kim TE, Smith DD Thoracic aortic dissection in an 18-year-old woman with no risk factors. *J Emerg Med.* 2010; 38(5):e41-e44.

33. Chen K, Varon J, Wenker OC, Judge DK, Fromm RE, Jr., Sternbach GL. Acute thoracic aortic dissection: The basics. *J Emerg Med.* 1997; 15(6):859-867.

34. Yam N, Lo CS, Ho CK. Acute aortic dissection associated with pregnancy. *Ann Thorac Surg.* 2015; 100(4):1470.

35. Zhu JM, Ma WG, Peterss S, Wang LF, Qiao ZY, Ziganshin BA et al. Aortic dissection in pregnancy: Management strategy and outcomes. *Ann Thorac Surg.* 2017; 103(4):1199-1206.

36. Shihata M, Pretorius V, MacArthur R. Repair of an acute type A aortic dissection combined with an emergency cesarean section in a pregnant woman. *Interact Cardiovasc Thorac Surg.* 2008; 7(5):938-940.

37. Morse BC, Boland BN, Morse JN, Jones YR, Simpson JP, Appleby DA et al. DeBakey type II aortic dissection: A rare catastrophic complication of pregnancy. *Am Surg.* 2014; 80(3):E79-E81.

38. Jovic TH, Aboelmagd T, Ramalingham G, Jones N, Nashef SA. Type A aortic dissection in pregnancy: Two operations yielding five healthy patients. *Aorta (Stamford).* 2014; 2(3):113-115.

39. Shu C, Fang K, Dardik A, Li X, Li M. Pregnancy-associated type B aortic dissection treated with thoracic endovascular aneurysm repair. *Ann Thorac Surg.* 2014; 97(2):582-587.

40. Gu X, Liu H, Li Y, Fei L, Shao D, Mao J et al. Spontaneous type B aortic dissection in antepartum gemellary pregnancy and endovascular repair. *Int J Clin Exp Med.* 2014; 7(11):4249-4252.

# 7

# *Hypoxemia*

**Lauren A. Plante, MD, MPH**

## CONTENTS

## Introduction and Background

In most cases, a clinical concern about hypoxemia stems from a reading generated by a peripheral device, the pulse oximeter. *Hypoxemia* itself is defined as a decrease in the partial pressure of oxygen in arterial blood ($P_aO_2$), while *hypoxia* refers to tissue oxygenation. Pulse oximetry does not measure either; it derives a measure of oxyhemoglobin saturation from the difference in the light absorption spectrum of oxyhemoglobin and deoxyhemoglobin (McMorrow and Mythen 2006). Signal strength requires a sufficient degree of pulsatile arterial blood flow, so in situations of compromised peripheral perfusion, pulse oximeter readings are unreliable. Other factors affecting accuracy are aberrant hemoglobins (fetal hemoglobin, erythrocyte sickling, carboxyhemoglobin, methemoglobin), intravenous dyes (methylene blue, indocyanine green), some nail polishes, and even certain types of lighting (fluorescent or xenon).

If the pulse oximetry shows a decreased saturation ($S_pO_2$), a bedside assessment of the patient is required. The patient's level of consciousness and respiratory effort should be quickly ascertained. Factors that might invalidate the pulse oximeter reading should be sought (movement artifact, decreased peripheral perfusion, hypothermia) before a decision is made to obtain arterial blood for analysis. Remember that the shape of the oxyhemoglobin saturation curve means that there may be significant differences in $P_aO_2$ at small differences in $S_pO_2$. Ninety-two percent is not close to 89%.

Arterial blood gas analysis provides a more reliable measure of oxygenation, although it is invasive and often painful.

A brief review of oxygenation follows. Inhaled gases are delivered to the alveoli, where a thin alveolar–capillary membrane and a huge surface area allow for rapid diffusion. The partial pressure of oxygen in inhaled air and in alveolar gas ($P_AO_2$) is much higher than the partial pressure of oxygen in mixed venous blood ($P_VO_2$) at the start of the pulmonary capillary, which drives oxygen uptake along the capillary until, by the end, the partial pressure of oxygen in the capillary ($P_{ec}O_2$) has nearly equilibrated with alveolar $P_AO_2$. Oxygen is transported in the blood either dissolved in plasma or bound to hemoglobin. Each gram of hemoglobin can bind 1.36 mL $O_2$ when fully saturated. Thus, arterial oxygen *content* is calculated as

$$C_aO_2 = 1.36 \times Hb \times S_aO_s/100 + 0.0031 \times P_aO_2.$$

It should be obvious that the contribution of dissolved oxygen is very small relative to the effect of hemoglobin. Oxygen *delivery* is the product of oxygen content and cardiac output.

## Causes of Hypoxemia

There are only five possible causes of hypoxemia. The first two are not clinically important in obstetric medicine.

1. Decreased fraction of inspired oxygen ($F_iO_2$) or partial pressure of inspired oxygen ($P_iO_2$)

    This is not relevant in clinical medicine. Pregnant women will seldom be subject to high enough altitude for this to be in the differential. (Inadvertent administration of hypoxic gas mixtures is no longer even possible with modern anesthesia machines or ventilators.)

2. Diffusion limitation

    This would apply in situations where either the alveolar–capillary membrane is thickened (for example, interstitial lung disease) or where the transit time of blood through pulmonary capillaries is so rapid that equilibration with alveolar $P_AO_2$ does not occur. This is seldom clinically relevant in obstetrics and does not happen in isolation regardless. It might contribute to hypoxemia in a patient in whom pulmonary blood flow is significantly increased and $P_iO_2$ is decreased, for example, high-level exercise at altitude or intersititial lung disease in the context of the higher cardiac output of pregnancy.

3. Hypoventilation

    Because hypoventilation decreases oxygen delivery but does not affect the A–a gradient, it easily corrects with supplemental oxygen. The decreased $P_aO_2$ (arterial) is a direct result of decreased $P_AO_2$ (alveolar) because inadequate ventilation reduces alveolar oxygenation. Hypoventilation may be central or neuromuscular, both of which may occur in obstetric patients. For example, opioid overdose depresses central respiratory drive. Too high a neuraxial block, or a neuromuscular condition such as myasthenia gravis, may affect respiratory muscle function. The direct clinical observation of respiratory rate and level of awareness are important tools in making this diagnosis, as is patient history. Note that periods of hypoventilation or apnea are especially likely to lead to oxygen desaturation in a pregnant woman, because oxygen demand is increased and functional residual capacity is decreased. $P_aCO_2$ is increased in hypoventilation.

4. Ventilation–perfusion (V/Q) mismatch

    This is a situation in which individual gas exchange units (alveolus with capillary) differ from one another with respect to ventilation, blood flow, or both. In the ideal lung, each gas exchange unit would have matched local ventilation and regional blood flow. However, a unit with inadequate ventilation (lower V/Q ratio) will have a local decrease in alveolar oxygenation, meaning that end-capillary blood leaving this unit will have a lower partial pressure of oxygen and therefore a lower oxygen content. The overall oxygen content of blood in the pulmonary circulation is related not to the partial pressure of oxygen from all these different units, but to their oxygen content. Since oxygen saturation cannot exceed 100% regardless of how high the local end-capillary partial pressure of oxygen is, the blood from highly ventilated units does not contribute additional oxygen content to the mixture leaving the pulmonary circulation, but blood from poorly ventilated units does lower the pooled content. The effect of V/Q mismatch is only in one direction. The A–a gradient (remember $P_aO_2$ is a composite) is increased. Some amelioration of hypoxemia can be achieved with supplemental oxygen.

    A lung unit with adequate ventilation but no perfusion represents dead space and cannot contribute to gas exchange. A lung unit with adequate ventilation but limited perfusion does not contribute much to gas exchange; blood flow is then redirected to other parts of the lung, which then manifest a locally decreased V/Q ratio.

    Examples of V/Q mismatch include pulmonary edema, atelectasis, chronic obstructive pulmonary disease, interstitial lung disease, and pneumonia.

5. Shunt

Shunts may be cardiac or intrapulmonary. While it is easy to visualize how intracardiac shunts give rise to systemic hypoxemia—by the admixture of deoxygenated blood with normally oxygenated blood—the concept of intrapulmonary shunt is not so apparent. Shunt may be understood as an extreme form of V/Q mismatch, where the amount of ventilation for a given lung unit is not just reduced but is zero. Since no gas exchange occurs in this unit, blood leaving the pulmonary capillary has the same oxygen content as blood that entered it. As mentioned earlier, this serves to reduce the overall arterial content. These areas will not correct with supplemental oxygen. The higher the shunt fraction (defined as the fraction of cardiac output perfusing nonventilated units), the worse the effect on arterial oxygenation and the less response to be expected from increasing $F_IO_2$. The A–a gradient is increased.

Intrapulmonary shunt may be due to pleural effusion, pulmonary arteriovenous malformation (rare), or acute respiratory distress syndrome (ARDS). One of the clinical criteria for ARDS is a severe impairment of oxygen exchange, manifested by a $P_aO_2/F_IO_2$ ratio less than 300. That is, on room air, $P_aO_2$ would be less than 63 mmHg, or less than 300 mmHg on 100% oxygen; compare this with normal numbers calculated from the alveolar gas equation (see Box 7.1).

When hypoxemia is confirmed, the initial therapeutic approach is to administer supplemental oxygen. Because the A–a gradient is widened when a pregnant woman is in a supine position, she should be moved to a sitting or semirecumbent position. Oxygen can be administered via a nasal cannula or via a

---

**BOX 7.1 CALCULATIONS: ALVEOLAR GAS EQUATION AND THE ALVEOLAR–ARTERIAL GRADIENT**

The alveolar gas equation is used to calculate the partial pressure of oxygen in the alveoli:

$$P_AO_2 = P_IO_2 - P_aCO_2/R = F_IO_2 \times (P_B - P_{H2O}) - P_aCO_2/R$$

Here the barometric pressure $P_B$ is either known or estimated based on the altitude; generally, at sea level, it is estimated as 760 mmHg. $P_{H2O}$ is the saturated vapor pressure of water, which is 47 mmHg at a temperature of 37°C. R is the respiratory quotient, which can be measured but is more commonly just assumed to be 0.8.

Thus, at sea level and at a normal body temperature of 37°C, with a measured $P_aCO_2$ of 40 mmHg, breathing room air with its $F_IO_2$ of 0.21 is

$$P_AO_2 = 0.21 \times (760 - 47) - 40/0.8 = 100 \text{ mmHg}$$

Similarly, one could calculate the $P_AO_2$ for a person breathing 100% $O_2$, that is, for $F_IO_2$ of 1.0,

$$P_AO_2 = 1 \times (760 - 47) - 40/0.8 = 663 \text{ mmHg}$$

The difference between the (calculated) $P_AO_2$ and the measured $P_aO_2$ in arterial blood is the alveolar–arterial difference, sometimes called the A–a gradient, or $P_{A-a}O_2$. Because gas exchange in the lung is not 100% efficient, there is a small difference, generally in the range of 2–6 mmHg. This does not change during pregnancy except to be affected by maternal position.

face mask. At a flow rate of 10 L/min, a nasal cannula delivers about 3 percentage points (above room air $F_1O_2$ of 21% or 0.21) per liter per minute flow rate. For example, a flow rate of 1 L/min would produce an $F_1O_2$ of approximately 0.24, and a flow rate of 5 L/min, about 0.36. (This varies some depending on the size of the patient's nasal cavity, since there is no other reservoir, and upon the respiratory demand, since higher demand entrains more room air.) A promising new development is the use of high-flow oxygen through a specialized system of nasal prongs (Optiflow™, Fisher & Paykel Healthcare), although as yet, there are no reports in pregnancy. Face masks can be fitted with a Venturi adapter, which can deliver different $F_1O_2$ between about 0.24 and 0.60, depending on the oxygen flow rate and the size of the entrainment port. Finally, a nonrebreather mask can deliver $F_1O_2$ between 0.60 and 0.90, depending on flow rates; these have both a reservoir bag inflated with oxygen and a series of one-way valves that prevent the entrainment of room air into the mask.

Hypoxemia due to hypoventilation easily corrects with supplemental $O_2$, so methods that deliver lower oxygen concentrations will usually be successful. Higher $F_1O_2$ will often be required for V/Q mismatch, depending on the degree of mismatch. Shunt will not correct well with supplemental $O_2$, unless the shunt fraction is very low indeed. This cause of hypoxemia will need additional interventions, such as non-invasive positive-pressure ventilation or intubation and mechanical ventilation.

A reasonable goal for oxygenation is to aim for maternal $P_aO_2$ above 60 mmHg, which corresponds to $S_aO_2$ above 90%. Below 90%, the oxyhemoglobin dissociation curve is steep. If the patient is unde-livered, there is often concern about fetal oxygenation, and many experts recommend maintaining $S_aO_2$ above 95%, but there is no clear evidence base for this recommendation, at least in humans. Fetal tissue oxygenation does not directly depend on maternal arterial oxygen content but on a combination of factors including maternal uterine venous oxygen content and placental perfusion. At appropriate gestational ages, the fetal heart rate tracing can be used as an indicator of the adequacy of fetal oxygenation when maternal hypoxemia is a concern.

The clinical assessment should occur concomitantly with the administration of oxygen. Primary eti-ologies of hypoxemia are cardiac vs. respiratory. Vital signs must be evaluated. Maternal respiratory rate is an indicator of respiratory drive: a low respiratory rate suggests an impairment of central drive, while a high rate indicates a compensatory response. (Apnea requires cardiopulmonary resuscitation or at least rescue ventilation.) Tachycardia may be a primary response to hypoxemia or may reflect infec-tion, pneumothorax, volume depletion, profound anemia, heart failure, or arrhythmia. Tachycardia is also a common sign of pulmonary embolus. Any irregular cardiac rhythm requires electrocardiogram assessment. Hypotension accompanies hypoxemia in amniotic fluid embolus, anaphylaxis, sepsis, pneu-mothorax (especially tension pneumothorax) and certain cardiac conditions. This escalates the level of urgency. Empiric treatment may be indicated if hypotension coexists with hypoxemia; address the most serious possible concern first.

The patient's level of consciousness should be assessed, as central nervous system (CNS) depression affects respiratory function. The recent administration of drugs (prescribed opioids or sedatives, or illic-itly obtained drugs) may be a factor. Urine toxicology is helpful in this context. The inability to carry on a conversation is a marker of significant compromise in an awake patient. The patient's position and the use of accessory muscles of respiration are clues as to her degree of respiratory effort.

Stridor indicates airway obstruction. Significant edema or jugular venous distension suggests heart failure, although mild degrees occur even in normal pregnancy. Auscultation of the heart and lungs must be performed. Although heart murmur is normal in pregnancy, it is usually a soft systolic murmur heard at the apex of the heart: anything else is pathological. Rales indicate pulmonary edema. Absent breath sounds suggest consolidation, e.g., pneumonia or pneumothorax or pleural effusion. Pneumothorax is typically painful and is more commonly traumatic or iatrogenic than spontaneous.

Wheezing is not pathognomonic of asthma or bronchospasm, but is a very common finding. Wheezing may also occur in other obstructive lung diseases, pulmonary embolus, and anaphylaxis and in vocal cord dysfunction.

After quick bedside assessment, laboratory testing and/or diagnostic imaging may be requested. ABG analysis is generally indicated, unless the patient is clearly hypoventilating due to CNS suppression, which will manifest as a slow respiratory rate. In that case, supplemental oxygen and a review of drugs admin-istered, with attention paid to whether they can be reversed (opioids via naloxone, benzodiazepines with flumazenil, etc.) is likely all that will be required. In all other cases, ABG provides information about the severity of hypoxemia, which can be quantitated by calculating the A–a gradient, and about the effectiveness of ventilation, measured from $P_aCO_2$. If the $P_aCO_2$ is normal or decreased, the ventilation is effective, while an increased $P_aCO_s$ means ineffective or failing ventilation. One frequent example is an elevated $P_aCO_2$ during asthma exacerbation, which means the patient's respiratory muscles are fatiguing and the next level of support should be considered. It is important to remember that the normal $P_aCO_2$ in pregnancy is 28–32 mmHg, so when the $P_aCO_s$ approaches 40 mmHg in a pregnant woman, this indicates ventilatory failure.

Chest X-ray can indicate cardiac or pulmonary pathology and may be done at the bedside if the patient is unstable for transport or if oxygenation cannot be maintained despite supplemental oxygen. Cardiomegaly, hyperinflation, pulmonary edema, pneumothorax, pleural effusion, and pneumonia are all easy to diagnose on a chest X-ray. Treatment should be directed toward the most likely cause.

If there is a clinical suspicion of pulmonary embolus, it is prudent to anticoagulate the patient while awaiting diagnostic testing. The cascade of testing will vary from institution to institution. Clinical suspicion plus abnormal lower extremity compression ultrasound studies are probably enough to assume pulmonary embolus, but negative lower extremity studies are insufficient to rule out pulmonary embolus: a V/Q scan or chest computed tomography (CT) scan will be required. The radiation burden is unequally distributed between these tests; the V/Q scan is associated with a higher fetal dose but a lower maternal dose than the chest CT. This translates into a slightly increased risk of childhood cancer for the infant with the V/Q scan and a somewhat higher risk of breast cancer for the mother with the chest CT. In practical terms, the testing strategy is usually determined by the institution's radiology guidelines. Either is acceptable.

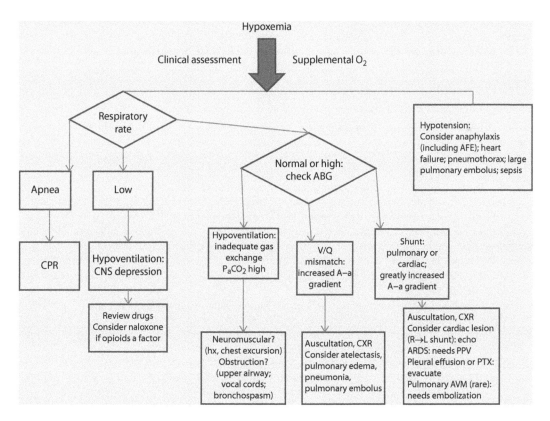

FIGURE 7.1 Algorithm for hypoxemia: administer $O_2$ while pursuing differential diagnosis. Depending on acuity, the treatment may be started on a clinical suspicion while a workup is ongoing (ABG, arterial blood gas; AFE, amniotic fluid embolus [also known as anaphylactoid syndrome of pregnancy]; AVM, arteriovenous malformation CNS, central nervous system; CPR, cardiopulmonary resuscitation; CXR, chest X-ray; $P_aCO_2$, partial pressure of oxygen in blood; R → L, right to left; V/Q, ventilation–perfusion).

ARDS is a clinical syndrome of profound hypoxemia coupled with bilateral opacities on chest imaging, not attributable to heart failure or fluid overload. The severity of oxygenation impairment is shown by the ratio of $P_aO_2/F_IO_2$, the cutoff for ARDS being less than 200. (Sample calculation: if $P_aO_2 = 200$ mmHg on $F_IO_2$ of 0.5, or 50%, the $P_aO_2/F_IO_2$ ratio is 400.) This is a nonspecific response of the lung, which may be precipitated by sepsis, trauma, burns, aspiration, transfusion, and many other factors. In obstetrics, it has been reported as a consequence of tocolytic drugs as well. ARDS requires positive-pressure ventilation, the application of positive end-expiratory pressure (PEEP), and high $F_IO_2$ to ameliorate hypoxemia. Although noninvasive positive-pressure ventilation systems have sometimes been proposed as a therapy, these are unsatisfactory in a pregnant patient, as they are uncomfortable and increase the risk of the aspiration of gastric contents. Intubation and mechanical ventilation is required. A system of high-flow oxygen therapy via specialized nasal cannula with the ability to provide both humidification and positive airway pressure (Optiflow) has been shown to decrease the need for intubation in nonpregnant adults with mild ARDS, but has not yet been evaluated in pregnancy.

A recurring question, which cannot be answered by existing evidence, is "What maternal $P_aO_2$ is required for fetal health?" Experts often recommend maintaining maternal $P_aO_2 > 60$ or 70 mmHg or $S_aO_2 > 90$ or >95%, voicing concerns about the potential for fetal hypoxia, but it is important to remember that the normal fetal state is one of hypoxemia not accompanied by tissue hypoxia. In most clinical situations, maternal oxygenation will be correctable with supplemental oxygen. In severe ARDS, this will not necessarily be true, of course, and the advent of lung-protective ventilator strategies often mean tolerating a degree of desaturation as low as 88% and/or a degree of respiratory acidosis as low as 7.15. A full discussion of fetal oxygen transport and the management of mechanical ventilation in pregnancy is beyond the scope of this chapter, however. Once the patient has been intubated and mechanical ventilation started (begin at $F_IO_2$ of 1.0, PEEP of 5 cm $H_2O$, and tidal volume of 6 mL/kg based on ideal body weight), she will be transferred to the intensive care unit (ICU). The interested reader should consult references on the management of the pregnant patient in the ICU for further details.

An algorithm for the diagnosis and treatment is given in Figure 7.1.

## SUGGESTED READING

ARDS Definition Task Force. Acute respiratory distress syndrome: The Berlin definition. *JAMA* 2012; 307:2526-2533.

Frat JP, Thille AW, Mercat A, Girault C, Ragot S et al. High-flow oxygen through nasal cannula in acute hypoxemic respiratory failure. *New Engl J Med* 2015; 372:2185-2196.

Lapinsky SE. Acute respiratory failure in pregnancy. *Obstet Med* 2015; 8:126-132.

Lapinsky SE, Rojas-Suarez JA, Crozier TM, Vasquez DN, Barrett N, Austin K et al. Mechanical ventilation in critically-ill pregnant women: a case series. *Int J Obstet Anest* 2015; 24:323-328.

Marik PE, Plante LA. Venous thromboembolic disease and pregnancy. *New Engl J Med* 2008; 359:2025-2033.

McMorrow RCN, Mythen MG. Pulse oximetry. *Curr Opin Critical Care* 2006; 12(3):269-271.

Mosier JM, Hypes C, Joshi R, Whitmore S, Parthasarathy S, Cairns CB. Ventilator strategies and rescue therapies for management of acute respiratory failure in the Emergency Department. *Ann Emerg Med* 2015; 66:529-541.

Petersson J and Glenny RW. Gas exchange and ventilation-perfusion relationships in the lung. *Eur Respir J* 2014; 44:1023-1041.

Pretto JJ, Roebuck T, Beckert L, Hamilton G. Clinical use of pulse oximetry: official guidelines from the Thoracic Society of Australia and New Zealand. *Respirology* 2014; 19:38-46.

Sarkar M, Niranjan N, Banyal PK. Mechanisms of hypoxemia. *Lung India* 2017; 34:47-60.

# 8

## Dyspnea

**Brigid McCue, MD, PhD**

Dyspnea, or shortness of breath, is a common complaint in pregnancy, reported by up to 70% of pregnant women. The American Thoracic Society defines dyspnea as "a subjective experience of breathing discomfort that consists of qualitatively distinct sensations that vary in intensity." The etiologies of dyspnea of pregnancy can be benign or life threatening, and rapid and effective triage is essential. This chapter will review the common causes of dyspnea and offer initial diagnostic and treatment options.

Physiological changes in pregnancy begin with fertilization and progress as the pregnancy develops. Multiple organ systems are affected by mechanical and hormonal adaptations to pregnancy. For instance, progesterone is a respiratory stimulant and induces an increase in $P_aO_2$ and a decrease in $P_aCO_2$ when administered to healthy, nonpregnant women and men (1). The elevation of the diaphragm by the gravid uterus reduces functional lung capacity and increases the "need to take a deep breath" often cited by women concerned about dyspnea on exertion. Oxygen consumption at rest is increased by 15–20% over nonpregnant women. Common physiological changes of pregnancy are summarized in Table 8.1 and shown graphically in Figure 8.1.

The most common etiology of shortness of breath in a pregnant patient is physiological dyspnea of pregnancy. Patients routinely complain of a reduced exercise tolerance for routine activities such as climbing stairs or talking on the phone. Sudden awakening or the abrupt need to gasp for breath can be caused by gastroesophageal reflux and relieved by antacids or interventions such as elevation of the head for sleep. The symptoms of physiological dyspnea of pregnancy have a gradual onset, peaking as the fundal height impinges on the diaphragm at 30–32 weeks, and do not cause significant disruption in activities of daily living. Patients display normal resting respiratory and heart rate and oxygen saturation of >92% on room air.

Routine adaptations of pregnancy can mask signs and symptoms of pathological dyspnea and increase susceptibility to the more dangerous etiologies of dyspnea. The hypercoagulability of pregnancy increases the risk of deep vein thrombosis (DVT) and pulmonary embolism (PE), increased venous return following delivery can unmask cardiac pathology, and pregnancy-specific pathologies such as amniotic fluid embolus complicate the workup for dyspnea of pregnancy. Suspicion must remain high for a pathological etiology despite the fact that the vast majority of complaints are benign.

The differential diagnosis for dyspnea in pregnancy includes those conditions that are specific to pregnancy, and those that cause dyspnea in the nonpregnant population such as airway, cardiac, and embolic disorders. Table 8.2 highlights the most common etiologies of dyspnea in pregnancy, diagnostic tests that should be considered, and initial therapies.

Of the nonphysiological causes of dyspnea in pregnancy, asthma is the most common, affecting 6–12% of pregnant women (2). Viral illness, postnasal drip, and symptoms of gastroesophageal reflux disease (GERD) exacerbate symptoms, and patients report that their usual asthma regimen is not as effective, or that their usual symptoms escalate more rapidly. Women with poor asthma control are at risk of miscarriage, prematurity, and intrauterine growth restriction (3). Spirometry is a reliable diagnostic tool in pregnancy (4). Medication management is similar to the nonpregnant patient, with the exception of systemic steroids, which may be associated with cleft palate in the first trimester (5). The overall safety of asthma medications for the fetus should be discussed with the patient before or soon after conception to encourage compliance. Acute exacerbations are aggressively managed with a low threshold for

TABLE 8.1

Physiological Changes in Pregnancy

| | | |
|---|---|---|
| *Pulmonary* | | |
| Respiratory rate | Unchanged | |
| Tidal volume | Increased 40% | |
| Functional residual capacity | Decreased 20% | |
| Vital capacity | Unchanged | |
| Minute ventilation | Increased 40% | |
| $O_2$ consumption | Increased 20–25% | |
| *Cardiac* | | |
| Heart rate | Increased 15% | |
| Cardiac output | Increased 30–50% | |
| Stroke volume | Increased | |
| Red blood cell mass | Increased 20–30% | |
| Plasma volume | Increased 40–50% | |
| Blood volume | Increased 50% | |
| Systemic blood pressure | Decreased 10–15 mmHg | Rises again after the second trimester |
| Pulmonary vascular resistance | Decreased | |
| Total peripheral resistance | Decreased 20% | |
| *Lab Values* | | |
| $P_aO_2$ (mmHg) | 80–104 | |
| $P_aCO_2$ (mmHg) | 30–32 | |
| Arterial (pH) | 7.40–7.48 | |
| Venous (pH) | 7.31–7.41 | |
| Bicarb (mEq/L) | 17.5–24.1 | |

noninvasive ventilation and/or intubation for unresponsive tachypnea or even a mildly elevated $P_aCO_2$ (6). Breastfeeding is encouraged to reduce the incidence of asthma in the offspring, and accommodation for breast pumping in the acute care setting is warranted.

Pregnant patients are more to susceptible to pneumonia, due to physiological changes such as altered immunity, increased oxygen consumption, restricted movement of the diaphragm, and risk of aspiration in labor and at the time of cesarean delivery. Pneumonia is the most common fatal nonobstetric infection in the pregnant patient (7). Pathogens are similar to those found in the nonpregnant patient, and include bacterial, viral, fungal, and mycobacterial agents, most likely community acquired. Varicella and influenza can be especially virulent in the pregnant population and are associated with an increased risk of morbidity and mortality (8,9). Medications to routinely avoid due to fetal effects include tetracyclines, sulfonamides, aminoglycosides, and quinolones. The threshold for a rapid response evaluation and admission to the critical care unit is lower for the pregnant patient, due to the potential for rapid deterioration and the dependency of the fetus on maternal oxygenation.

Pregnancy and the postpartum period are risk factors for venous thromboembolus, with an incidence estimated at 0.76–1.72 per 1000 pregnancies (10). Presenting symptoms include dyspnea, chest pain, fatigue, and palpitations, with or without symptoms of DVT. Vital signs can be normal or show varying degrees of maternal tachycardia, hypotension, and hypoxia. A useful algorithm for the diagnostic workup of pulmonary embolism in pregnancy is presented by Leung et al. (11) (Figure 8.2) and suggests initial Doppler ultrasound of the lower extremities, chest X-ray (CXR) followed by ventilation–perfusion (V/Q) scan in the absence of lung pathology and computed-tomographic pulmonary angiography if the CXR demonstrates lesions likely to result in an indeterminate V/Q scan. Treatment is recommended if

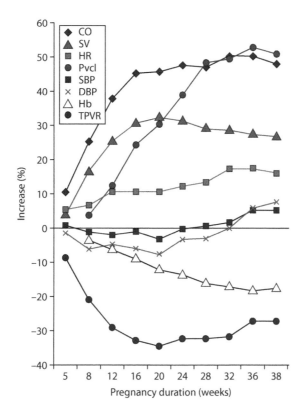

FIGURE 8.1 Changes in CO, PV, HR, SV, TPVR, SBP, DBP, and Hb during pregnancy. (Data from Robson, S. C. et al., *American Journal of Physiology*, 256, H1060–H1065, 1989; reprinted from *American Journal of Obstetrics and Gynecology*, 170, Mabie, W. C. et al., A longitudinal study of cardiac output in normal human pregnancy, 849–56, Copyright (1994), with permission from Elsevier.) CO, cardiac output; DBP, diastolic blood pressure; Hb, hemoglobin concentration; HR, heart rate; PV, plasma volume; SV, stroke volume; SBP, systolic blood pressure; TPVR, total peripheral vascular resistance. (From Karamermer, Y., and Roos-Hesselink, J. W., *Expert Review of Cardiovascular Therapy*, 5, 859–69, 2007. With permission.)

a positive result is obtained at any point in the workup. Cardiac echo can be considered if a large pulmonary embolus resulting in hemodynamic instability is suspected, but is not sensitive for small emboli (12).

The treatment of pulmonary embolus in the stable pregnant patient is anticoagulation to limit clot extension, either with heparin or low-molecular-weight formulations. Subcutaneous dosing can begin with enoxaparin 1 mg/kg Q for 12 hours and titrate to an anti-Xa level of 0.6–1.0 IU/mL U. After the appropriate dose is determined, continued measurement of anti-Xa levels is not recommended (13).

Patients at a high risk of bleeding, for delivery, or who are clinically unstable, should receive anti-coagulation with intravenous (IV) unfractionated heparin at a bolus of 80 units/kg followed by a continuous infusion of 18 units/kg titrating to a therapeutic activated prothrombin time and transitioned to subcutaneous heparin in 5–10 days (14). Patients therapeutically anticoagulated are not candidates for regional anesthesia due to the risk of spinal hematoma. Anticoagulation can be resumed 6 hours after a vaginal birth and 12 hours after a cesarean birth. The American Society for Reproductive Medicine recommends the resumption of either heparin or low-molecular weight heparin 2 hours after the removal of an epidural catheter, with a longer interval considered in the event of traumatic placement (15). The duration of therapy postpartum should be individualized.

The safety of thrombolytic therapy in pregnancy has not been established, but case reports demonstrate success and could be considered for the hemodynamically unstable patient as a life-saving intervention. One review of case reports of 172 pregnant women treated with thrombolytic agents

TABLE 8.2

Common Etiologies of Dyspnea, Diagnosis, and Treatment Options

| | Symptoms and Risk Factors | Testing | Interventions |
|---|---|---|---|
| Changes in pregnancy | Gradual onset, mild | H+P, PE | Reassurance |
| GERD | Associated with poor oral intake | H+P, PE | Antacids, non-pharmacologic measures |
| Anxiety/panic | Sudden onset, feeling of doom | H+P, PE | Therapy, SSRI/SNRI |
| *Pulmonary* | | | |
| Asthma | Chest tightness/wheezing; Exercise/viral syndrome; More rapid exacerbations than in pre-pregnancy | Spirometry | Beta-agonists, steroids, maintenance medications, $O_2$ supplement |
| Pneumonia | Fever, cough, chest pain; sudden onset; Associated with viral syndrome, aspiration | Shielded CXR | Antibiotics, beta-agonists, $O_2$ supplement, CCU consultation |
| Pulmonary edema | Sudden onset; IV fluids, tocolysis, multiple gestation; Tachycardia, tachypnea, and low $O_2$ saturation | Shielded CXR | Diuresis |
| Pulmonary embolus | Sudden onset, chest/abdominal pain, ± DVT; Tachycardia, low index suspicion | LE Dopplers, V/Q vs CT-A | Anticoagulation, consider thrombolysis |
| AFE | Emergent onset, disorientation; Hypotension, DIC, respiratory collapse | Cardiac echo | ECMO |
| *Cardiac* | | | |
| Arrhythmia | Sudden onset, palpations, dizziness | ECG, Holter monitor | Beta-blocker, Ca channel blocker |
| MI | Chest/abdominal pain, nausea; Obesity, AMA, DM | Serial enzymes; ECG | Cardiac catheterization, stent |
| Cardiomyopathy | Gradual onset, edema; Postpartum, paroxysmal nocturnal dyspnea | Cardiac echo, ECG | Manage heart failure; Consult cardiology |
| Aortic/coronary dissection | Sudden onset chest pain; Marfan syndrome | Cardiac echo, ECG | Control hypertension, arrhythmia; Consult cardiothoracic surgeon |

*Note:* AMA, advanced maternal age; Ca, calcium; CCU, critical care unit; CTA, computed tomography angiography; CXR, chest X-ray; DM, diabetes mellitus; DVT, deep vein thrombosis; ECG, electrocardiogram; H+P, history and physical; IV, intravenous; LE, lower extremities; MI, myocardial infarction; $O_2$, oxygen; PE, physical exam; SSNI, serotonin-norepinephrine reuptake inhibitor; SSRI, selective serotonin reuptake inhibitor; V/Q, ventilation–perfusion scan.

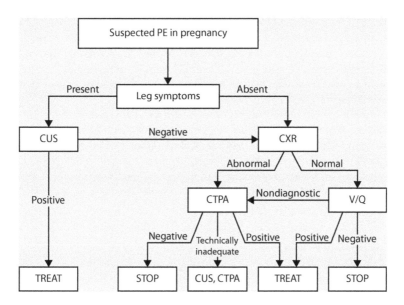

**FIGURE 8.2** Algorithm for suspected pulmonary embolism in pregnancy. (Reprinted from Leung, A. N. et al., *American Journal of Respiratory and Critical Care Medicine*, 184, 1200–1208, 2011. With permission.)

found a maternal mortality of 1%, incidence of fetal loss of 6%, and incidence of maternal hemorrhage of 8% (16). Thrombectomy and inferior vena cava filters have also been reported effective in pregnancy.

Amniotic fluid embolus is a clinical diagnosis, which classically presents with acute dyspnea, hypoxia, hypotension, change in mental status, and disseminated intravascular coagulation (differentiating amniotic fluid embolus from pulmonary embolus). The incidence of amniotic fluid embolism (AFE) ranges from 1 to 12 per 100,000, and risk factors include uterine trauma (cesarean delivery, operative vaginal delivery, miscarriage, abortion and cervical laceration, placenta previa or accreta), advanced maternal age, and grand multiparity (17). The etiology is unknown but is presumed to involve amniotic fluid entering the maternal circulation causing cardiogenic shock, respiratory collapse, and anaphylactoid reaction. AFE syndrome is unpredictable and unpreventable.

The treatment of AFE is cardiovascular support with oxygenation, IV fluids, blood products, vasopressors, and inotropic agents and requires a multidisciplinary team approach. Hemodynamic monitoring with central lines is essential to monitor volume status and prevent pulmonary edema. Disseminated intravascular coagulopathy (DIC) complicates 83% of the cases of AFE, and massive transfusion protocols are often activated to adequately replace blood products (18). When available, bedside thromboelastography may identify patients who might benefit from antifibrinolytics such as tranexamic acid (19). The successful use of extracorporeal membrane oxygenation (ECMO), lipid emulsion rescue, and inhaled nitric oxide have been described in case reports (20,21). Although current management has reportedly reduced maternal mortality to 20%, there remains an 85% incidence of neurological injury among survivors (22).

Additional etiologies for dyspnea that present with more than simple dyspnea such as primary pulmonary hypertension, restrictive lung disease such as sarcoid, and genetic diseases such as cystic fibrosis will not be discussed here.

Cardiac disease in pregnancy and the postpartum period can also present with dyspnea and was the most common cause of maternal mortality seen in a recent review (23). The majority of deaths occurred in women with structurally normal hearts, who were not previously diagnosed with cardiac disease. Care was deemed substandard in >50% of the patients due to failure to investigate chest pain and inadequate evaluation for ischemia. The immediate postpartum period remains the highest risk for cardiac dysfunction, due to the increased venous return following the release of vena cava compression, uterine and placental autotransfusion, and IV fluid overload during labor management.

Hemodynamic changes of pregnancy begin in the first trimester, with cardiac output increased by 50% by the second trimester and reaching a peak during the metabolic demands of labor (see Figure 8.1). The increased venous return immediately following delivery can unmask ventricular dysfunction and persist for several weeks postpartum. All women with identified cardiac disease should use contraception and seek preconception counsel regarding the risk of a pregnancy to the mother and potential child. Thorne et al. (24) classified maternal risk by lesion, summarized in Table 8.3.

Palpitations are a common complaint in pregnancy due to atrial or ventral ectopy, exacerbated by fluid shifts. Palpitations are generally benign, unless they are associated with sustained symptoms, dizziness, dyspnea, or chest pain, which may be an early indication of ventricular dysfunction. Arrhythmia on electrocardiogram (ECG) should prompt an echocardiogram to rule out impaired ventricular function. Symptomatic palpitations not due to structural lesions can be managed with beta-blockers, adequate hydration, and avoidance of caffeinated beverages.

## TABLE 8.3

Classification of Maternal Risk by Lesion[a]

| *Class I* (no detectable increase in maternal mortality and no or mild increase in morbidity) | *Class II* (small increase in maternal mortality and moderate increase in morbidity) | *Classes II and III* | *Class III* (significantly increased risk of maternal mortality or severe morbidity) | *Class IV* (extremely high risk of maternal mortality or severe morbidity) |
|---|---|---|---|---|
| Uncomplicated small or mild: | Unoperated ASD | Mild left ventricular impairment | Mechanical valve | Pulmonary hypertension of any cause |
| • Pulmonary stenosis<br>• VSD<br>• PDA<br>• Mitral valve prolapse | Repaired tetralogy of Fallot | Hypertrophic cardiomyopathy | Systemic right ventricle | Severe systemic ventricular impairment—LVEF is <30% or NYHA III–IV |
| | Most arrhythmias | Native or tissue valve disease not considered class IV | • CCTGA | Previous peripartum cardiomyopathy with any residual ventricular impairment |
| | | Marfan syndrome (or other aortopathy, e.g., EDS type IV, LDS, or FTAA) without aortic dilatation | • TGA with Mustard or Senning repair | Severe left heart obstruction |
| | | Repaired coarctation | Post-Fontan repair | Marfan's syndrome with aorta >45 mm |
| Successfully repaired simple lesions, e.g.,<br><br>Secundum ASD, VSD, PDA, total anomalous pulmonary venous drainage | | Heart transplantation | Cyanotic heart disease<br><br>Other complex congenital heart disease | |
| | | | Marfan syndrome with aorta 40–45 mm | |

*Source:*  Thorne, S. et al., *Heart*, 92, 1520–1525, 2006.

*Note:*  ASD, atrial septal defect; CCTGA, congenitally corrected transposition of the great arteries; EDS, Ehlers-Danlos syndrome; FTAA, familial thoracic aortic aneurysm; LDS, Loeys-Dietz syndrome; LVEF, left ventricular ejection fraction; NYHA, New York Heart Association; PDA, patent ductus arteriosus; TGA, transposition of the great arteries; VSD, ventricular septal defect.

[a]  See further Thorne et al. (24) for data.

The incidence of coronary artery disease (CAD) is increasing in the pregnant population, due to changing demographics regarding advanced maternal age and increasing incidence of obesity and diabetes. A review of maternal mortality in the UK identified CAD as the etiology in 20% of cases of maternal mortality (25). The sometimes atypical presentation of ischemia in women and the overlap of routine discomforts of pregnancy, such as epigastric pain, dyspnea, and heart palpitations, resulted in inadequate evaluation in 46% of women in the UK study who died of CAD. Suspicion for cardiac disease should remain high, and ECG and serial troponins remain reliable in pregnancy.

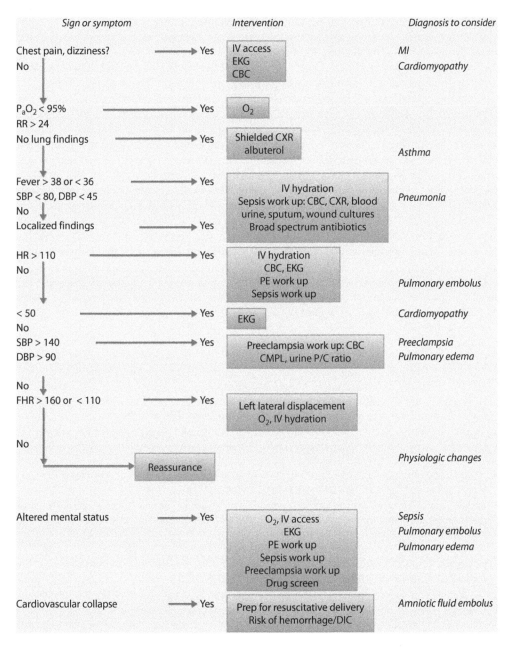

FIGURE 8.3 Dyspnea algorithm: a patient presents with shortness of breath in pregnancy. CBC, complete blood count; CMPL, comprehensive metabolic panel and liver function tests; FHR, fetal heart rate; HR, heart rate; P/C, protein/creatinine ratio; RR, respiratory rate; SBP, systolic blood pressure.

The treatment of ST elevation and non-ST elevation myocardial infarction (MI) is similar in pregnant or nonpregnant patients, with emergent coronary angiography and primary percutaneous coronary intervention as indicated. Due to the increased flow within the femoral veins, radial access is preferred, and abdominal lead shield and pelvic tilt are essential to minimize fetal risk. Medical therapy with beta-blockade and low-dose aspirin is considered safe in pregnancy.

Peripartum cardiomyopathy occurs with an incidence of 4.84 per 10,000 live births, in the last few months of pregnancy or up to 5 months postpartum (26). Risk factors include preeclampsia, history of cardiomyopathy, history of chemotherapy treatment, advanced maternal age, and multiparity (27). Symptoms such as dyspnea and pedal edema may have an insidious onset and be attributed to normal pregnancy complaints. Maternal mortality is 15–30%, with recurrence in subsequent pregnancies of 20–40% (28). Medical management is similar to nonpregnant patients, and anticoagulation is generally indicated due to the risk of intracardiac thrombus formation.

The safety profiles of cardiac medications vary in pregnancy and lactation, and some have negative fetal effects. Beta-blockers may be associated with fetal growth restriction and should prompt serial growth scans. Angiotensin-converting enzyme inhibitors, angiotensin receptor blockers, and angiotensin receptor–neprilysin inhibitors are contraindicated as they are associated with oligohydramnios, fetal death, and neonatal renal failure after delivery, but may be considered for the breastfeeding mother (29). Vasodilation can be safely achieved during pregnancy with hydralazine and nitrates. Loop diuretics should replace aldosterone antagonists due the feminization of the male fetus. Digoxin may be considered for patients with symptoms resistant to diuresis and vasodilator therapy (30).

Resuscitation in pregnancy requires modification due to physiological and hemodynamic changes of pregnancy and the presence of the fetus. Such modifications include uterine displacement (if the fundus is at or above the umbilicus), placement of IV access above the diaphragm, proactive management of the airway, and consideration of the resuscitative hysterotomy to save the fetus and to facilitate resuscitation of the mother (31). Defibrillation may proceed at the usual energy levels, after the removal of the fetal monitoring devices. Diagnostic imaging should proceed with abdominal shielding, when possible.

In summary, dyspnea is most commonly a benign symptom of pregnancy, but effective and timely triage of the pregnant patient is necessary to ensure that significant pulmonary or cardiac disease is properly diagnosed and treated. See Figure 8.3.

## REFERENCES

1. Skatrud JB, Dempsey JA, Kaiser DG. Ventalatory response to medroxyprogesterone acetate in normal subjects: Time course and mechanism. *J Appl Physiol Respir Environ Exerc Physiol.* 1978; 44(6):939-944.
2. Kwon HL, Triche EW, Belanger K, Bracken MB. The epidemiology of asthma during pregnancy; prevalence, diagnosis and symptoms. *Immunol Clin North Am.* 2006; 26(1):29-62.
3. Tata LJ, Lewis SA, McKeever TM, Smith CJ, Doyle P, Smeeth L et al. A comprehensive analysis of adverse obstetric and pediatric complications in women with asthma. *Am J Respir Crit Care Med.* 2007; 175(10):991-997.
4. Hirnle L, Lysenko L, Gerber H, Lesnik P, Baranowska A, Rachwalik M et al. Respiratory function in pregnant women. *Adv Exp Med Biol.* 2013; 788:153-160.
5. Park-Wyllie L, Mazzotta P, Pastuszak A, Moretti ME, Beique L, Hunnisett L et al. Birth defects after maternal exposure to corticosteroids: A prospective cohort study and meta-analysis of epidemiological studies. *Tetrology.* 2000; 62(6):385-392.
6. Mighty HE. Acute respiratory failure in pregnancy. *Clin Obstet Gynecol.* 2010; 53(2):360-368.
7. Creanga AA, Berg CJ, Syverson C, Seed K, Bruce FC, Callaghan WM. Pregnancy-related mortality in the United States, 2006–2010. *Obstet Gynecol.* 2015; 125(1):5-12.
8. Callaghan WM, Chu SY, Jamieson DJ. Deaths from seasonal influenza among pregnant women in the United States, 1998–2005. *Obstet Gynecol.* 2010; 115(5):919-923.
9. Harger JH, Ernest JM, Thurnau GR, Moawad A, Momirova V, Landon MB et al. Risk factors and outcomes of varicella-zoster virus pneumonia in pregnant women. *J Infect Dis.* 2002; 185(4):422-427.
10. Marik PE, Plante LA. Venous thromboembolic disease and pregnancy. *N Engl J Med.* 2008; 359(19): 2025-2033.

11. Leung AN, Bull TM, Jaeschke R, Lockwood CJ, Boiselle PM, Hurwitz LM et al. An official American Thoracic Society/Society of Thoracic Radiology clinical practice guideline: Evaluation of suspected pulmonary embolism in pregnancy. *Am J Respir Crit Care Med.* 2011; 184(10):1200-1208.
12. Pavan D, Nicolosi GL, Antonini-Canterin F, Zanuttini D. Echocardiography in pulmonary embolism disease. *Int J Cardiol.* 1998; 65(Suppl 1):S87-S90.
13. Bates SM, Greer IA, Middeldorp S, Veenstra DL, Prabulos AM, Vandvik PO et al. VTE, thrombophilia, antithrombotic therapy, and pregnancy: Antithrombotic therapy and prevention of thrombosis, 9th ed: American College of Chest Physicians Evidence-Based Clinical Practice Guidelines. *Chest.* 2012; 141(2 Suppl):e691S.
14. Toglia MR, Weg JG. Venous thromboembolism during pregnancy. *N Engl J Med.* 1996; 335(2):108-114.
15. Horlocker TT, Wedel DJ, Rowlingson JC, Enneking FK, Kopp SL, Benzon HT et al. Regional anesthesia in the patient receiving antithrombotic or thrombolytic therapy: American Society of Regional Anesthesia and Pain Medicine Evidence-Based Guidelines (Third Edition). *Reg Anesth Pain Med.* 2010; 35(1):64-101.
16. Turrentine MA, Braems G, Ramirez MM. Use of thrombolytics for the treatment of thromboembolic disease during pregnancy. *Obstet Gynecol Surv.* 1995; 50(7):534-541.
17. Abenhaim HA, Azoulay L, Kramer MS, Leduc L. Incidence and risk factors of amniotic fluid embolisms: A population-based study on 3 million births in the United States. *Am J Obstet Gynecol.* 2008; 199(1):49.e1-8.
18. Clark SL, Hankins GD, Dudley DA, Dildy GA, Porter TF. Amniotic fluid embolism: Analysis of the national registry. *Am J Obstet Gynecol.* 1995; 172:1158-1169.
19. Collins NF, Bloor M, McDonnell NJ. Hyperfibrinolysis diagnosed by rotational thromboelastography in a case of suspected amniotic fluid embolism. *Int J Obstet Anesth.* 2013; 22:71-76.
20. Ecker JL, Solt K, Fitzsimons MG, MacGillivray TE. Case records of the Massachusetts General Hospital: Case 40-2012: A 43-year-old woman with cardiorespiratory arrest after a cesarean section. *N Engl J Med.* 2012; 367(26):2528-2536.
21. Lynch W, McAllister RK, Lay JF, Jr., Culp WC, Jr. Lipid emulsion rescue of amniotic fluid embolism-induced cardiac arrest: A case report. *AA Case Rep.* 2017; 8(3):64-66.
22. Berg CJ, Callaghan WM, Syverson C, Henderson Z. Pregnancy-related mortality in the United States, 1998 to 2005. *Obstet Gynecol.* 2010; 116(6):1302-1309.
23. Main EK, McCain CL, Morton CH, Holtby S, Lawton ES. Pregnancy-related mortality in California: Causes, characteristics, and improvement opportunities. *Obstet Gynecol.* 2015; 125:938-947.
24. Thorne S, MacGregor A, Nelson-Piercy C. Risks of contraception and pregnancy in heart disease. *Heart.* 2006; 92(10):1520-1525.
25. Cantwell R, Clutton-Brock T, Cooper G, Dawson A, Drife J, Garrod D et al. Saving Mother's Lives: Reviewing maternal deaths to make motherhood safer: 2006–2008. *BJOG.* 2011; 118:1-203.
26. Gunderson EP, Croen LA, Chiang V, Yoshida CK, Walton D, Go AS. Epidemiology of peripartum cardiomyopathy: Incidence, predictors and outcomes. *Obstet Gynecol.* 2011; 118(3):583-591.
27. Sliwa K, Hilfiker-Kleiner D, Petrie MC, Mebazaa A, Pieske B, Buchmann E et al. Current state of knowledge on aetiology, diagnosis, management and therapy of peripartum cardiomyopathy: A position statement from the Heart Failure Association of the European Society of Cardiology Working Group on Peripartum Cardiomyopathy. *Eur J Heart Fail.* 2014; 12(8):767-778.
28. Elkayam U, Jalnapurkar S, Barakat M. Peripartum cardiomyopathy. *Cardiol Clin.* 2012; 30(3):435-440.
29. Shotan A, Widerhorn J, Hurst A, Elkayam U. Risks of angiotensin-converting enzyme inhibition during pregnancy: Experimental and clinical evidence, potential mechanisms and recommendations for use. *Am J Med.* 1994; 96(5):451-456.
30. Regitz-Zagrosek V, Blomstrom Lundqvist C, Borghi C, Cifkova R, Ferreira R, Foidart JM et al. European Society of Gynecology, Association for European Paediatric Cardiology, German Society for Gender Medicine et al. ESG guidelines on the management of cardiovascular diseases during pregnancy: The Task Force on Management of Cardiovascular Diseases during Pregnancy of the European Society of Cardiology (ESC). *Eur Heart J.* 2011; 32:3147-3197.
31. Jeejeebhoy FM, Zelop CM, Lipman S et al. Cardiac arrest in pregnancy: A scientific statement from the American Heart Association. *Circulation.* 2015; 132(18):1747-1773.

# 9

## Oliguria

**Jhenette Lauder, MD and Anthony Sciscione, DO**

### CONTENTS

## Introduction

Oliguria is defined as an abnormal and sustained low urine output (UOP). It occurs as a result of some kind of renal compromise. In most instances, this does not involve permanent damage to the renal parenchyma and is easily reversible with conservative interventions like fluid hydration.

In the obstetric patient, oliguria is often a transient aberration and a reflection of acute and self-limited insults to the renal system. In this patient population, the mechanism of action is primarily due to renal hypoperfusion with impaired autoregulation, which is termed *prerenal acute kidney injury* (AKI). The most common etiologies in pregnancy include hypovolemia from hemorrhage or hypertensive disorders causing renal vasospasm. In addition, in critical clinical scenarios, such as preeclampsia (PEC) with severe features, severe sepsis, and hypovolemic shock, oliguria is a reflection of the severity of the underlying disease process and serves as a clinical sign of end organ damage.

In this chapter, we will review the renal physiology in pregnancy, the definition and pathophysiology of oliguria, the differential diagnosis of AKI within the obstetric patient and its diagnostic workup, and the specific management approaches for its various etiologies.

## Definition of Oliguria

Oliguria is defined as a urine output rate less than 0.5 cm$^3$/kg/hour. Oliguria can also be defined in more general terms as a UOP rate less than 30 cm$^3$/hour or less than 400 cm$^3$ in a 24-hour period in the average body mass index (BMI) patient (1). However, in the obese patient, these alternative definitions can be deceivingly reassuring. Accounting for a patient's weight is imperative in these instances to have an accurate understanding of the clinical picture at hand (see Table 9.1).

Furthermore, true oliguria is thought to be sustained over the course of 4–6 hours and does not readily respond to fluids. In addition, it is usually associated with an elevated serum creatinine (sCRT)—another clinical sign of renal comprise. In the absence of known kidney disease, oliguria and an elevated

TABLE 9.1

Oliguria: Clinical Parameters

| Urine output that is below |
| --- |
| • 0.5 mL/kg/hour for at least 4–6 hours |
| • Less than 400 mL in 24 hours |
| • Less than 30 mL/hour |

creatinine often acutely occur in healthy obstetric patients following a well-defined insult, such as a significant postpartum hemorrhage.

## Renal Physiology and Pathophysiology in Pregnancy

The structure and functional capacity of the kidneys changes significantly during pregnancy and can be first appreciated as early as 6 weeks of gestation. In simple terms, the kidneys "rev up" in size and performance to accommodate the metabolic demands required to support a growing fetus and placenta. For example, the parenchyma, including its collecting system, increases in size and dilates to accommodate the increase in blood volume and cardiac output that occurs during pregnancy (2).

In addition, systematic vasodilation leads to an increase in renal blood flow by as much as 50–85% and an increase in glomerular filtration rate (GFR) by 40–65% (1). As a result, there is a decrease in sCRT and blood urea nitrogen (BUN) levels. When assessing for signs of renal compromise in a pregnant patient, changes in renal physiology must be taken into account, and the normal ranges, adjusted to reflect these changes. In pregnancy, the normal creatinine level changes to <0.8 mg/dL, and similarly the BUN becomes <8.0 mg/dL (1,3,4) (Table 9.2). However, despite this increase in size and activity, the kidneys' metabolic processes and feedback loops remain unchanged in pregnancy.

In the obstetric population, oliguria is most commonly a clinical manifestation of an acute compromise of the renal compensatory response to hypoperfusion. This is commonly classified as prerenal AKI.

In the presence of decreased perfusion, there is a well-defined autoregulation process that occurs in the kidney. First, a decrease in blood flow stimulates the release of local prostaglandins, which results in the vasodilatation of the afferent arterioles. As a result, there is an increase in blood volume entering the glomerular system. In addition, there is concomitant vasoconstriction of the efferent arterioles, due to the release of angiotensin II. This leads to an increase in the glomerular hydrostatic pressure. The combination of both processes allows for the maintenance of the GFR pressure, which results in a sustained glomerular filtration and the excretion of nitrogenous waste products, as well as creatinine (5).

The kidney, in an attempt to restore volume, reabsorbs more water than usual from the renal tubules, while continuing to excrete waste products in concentrated urine. As is expected, the urine volume in this setting is low. If the hypoperfusion is addressed early, for instance with fluid hydration, the restoration of intravascular volume will dampen the renal autoregulation processes in a negative feedback loop. Urine then becomes more dilute and increases in volume.

However, in the presence of prolonged hypoperfusion and/or exposure to medications that disrupt this autoregulation process, such as nonsteroidal anti-inflammatory drugs (NSAIDs), angiotensin-converting enzyme inhibitors (ACEis), or angiotensin receptor blockers (ARBs), this compensatory response becomes dysregulated (5). GFR decreases, leading to an intravascular buildup in nitrogenous waste products, an elevated sCRT, and oliguria. This breakdown of renal autoregulation defines prerenal AKI.

TABLE 9.2

Creatinine Variations

| Normal pregnancy values: |
| --- |
| • Creatinine: <0.8 mg/dL |
| • BUN: <8.0 mg/dL |
| AKI: |
| • Creatinine: ↑ by at least 0.3 mg/dL *or* ↑ by 50% from prior baseline |

## Acute Kidney Injury

AKI is an acute insult to the renal system that results in a loss of normal renal function. It can be objectively measured as an elevation in sCRT and BUN or the acute onset of oliguria. More specifically, it is clinically defined as an elevation in creatinine by at least 0.3 mg/dL or an increase in baseline by 50% or more (5) (Table 9.2). In most clinical scenarios, AKI is self-limiting with a full return of renal function. Very rarely in the developing world do obstetric patients require renal replacement therapy as a result of complications of AKI.

AKI is a clinical phenomenon that can occur as a result of various etiologies. Traditionally, it is understood to be a result of one of three distinct pathophysiological pathways: prerenal azotemia, intrinsic renal injury, or postrenal injury (5). Each subset of AKI has unique etiologies (see Figure 9.1). As previously discussed, the former is a result of renal hypoperfusion; the etiology of which can vary, but includes hypovolemia and acute worsening of hypertension (HTN). Additionally, in the obstetric patient, prerenal azotemia is the most likely culprit of AKI and thus oliguria (3).

Prerenal AKI, itself, does not specifically cause parenchymal damage. However, if the underlying insult persists, eventually, tissue injury will largely occur as a result of prolonged ischemia. The most common manifestation of this injury is acute tubular necrosis or, in severe cases, acute cortical necrosis.

In contrast, intrinsic AKI does involve some level of tissue damage and can affect all areas of renal anatomy depending on the etiology, including tubule or interstitial cells; the glomerular matrix; or vasculature. As such, the resolution of intrinsic AKI may be more prolonged, even in healthy obstetric patients. However, it does not generally result in long-standing sequelae when promptly addressed. The most common etiologies in the pregnant patient include sepsis; ischemia from prolonged hypoperfusion or HTN; and common nephrotoxins, including antibiotics (vancomycin, aminoglycosides) and imaging contrast.

Lastly, postrenal AKI is a result of obstruction at any point in the genitourinary system, including the bladder, ureters, and renal pelvis. It is a relatively uncommon cause of oliguria in healthy populations. In the presence of two normally functioning kidneys, obstruction must be bilateral for a clinical manifestation of postrenal AKI. For example, in the obstetric patient, the growing uterus is known to cause mild hydronephrosis, primarily on the right side, due to the mechanical obstruction of the ureter at the pelvic

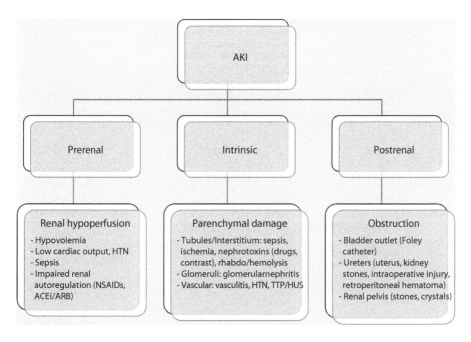

**FIGURE 9.1** AKIs: etiologies.

prim. However, this does not generally cause clinical AKI in isolation (2). More common etiologies include obstructing nephrolithiasis, impacted Foley catheter, or ureteral injury during cesarean section.

## Differential Diagnosis for Oliguria

When approaching the differential diagnosis of oliguria, it is important to consider the gestational age at the time of presentation (Figure 9.2). The common causes of oliguria will vary depending on a patient's trimester (1). For example, in the first trimester, oliguria most commonly occurs in the setting of prolonged hypotension from either hypovolemia or septic cardiovascular collapse. Hypovolemia may occur due to the gastrointestinal insensible losses sustained in cases of hyperemesis gravidarum or severe cases of gastroenteritis. It may also be a reflection of acute blood loss in the setting of a spontaneous abortion (SAB) following expectant management or medical/surgical intervention. In most instances, severe hemorrhage from SAB is related to retained products of conception (POCs).

The cardiovascular collapse or hypotension seen in severe sepsis can also lead to oliguria and, in the first trimester, is most commonly a result of septic abortion or infections of the respiratory or genitourinary system. Additionally, bacterial and viral infections in pregnancy are known to be far more severe than those in the nonpregnant patient and more often result in hospitalization.

An uncommon but significant reason for oliguria/anuria in the first or early second trimester of pregnancy is due to a uterine incarceration. In this entity, a significantly retroverted and/or retroflexed uterus becomes impacted in the pelvis and obstructs the urethra.

The differential diagnosis for the latter trimesters and postpartum period includes more obstetrically related conditions, which are also generally more common. For example, intrauterine and postpartum hemorrhage are likely the most common causes of oliguria worldwide. The common etiologies of intrauterine bleeding include placenta previa and placental abruption. Uterine rupture is less so but is potentially catastrophic for both mother and fetus when it does occur.

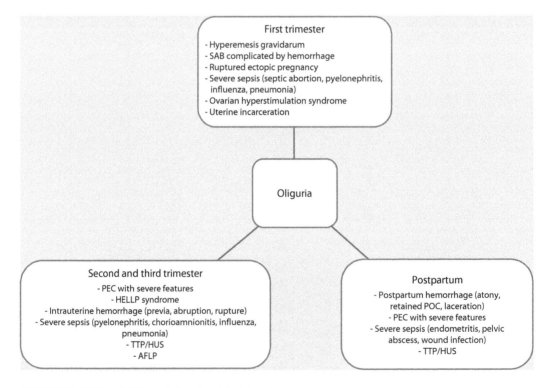

FIGURE 9.2   Differential diagnosis for oliguria by trimesters.

Postpartum hemorrhage often presents in the setting of uterine atony. However, retained placenta or membranes and cervical or perineal lacerations are also important etiologies of massive maternal blood loss. Oliguria, or more generally AKI, occurs following these events in the setting of inadequate or untimely resuscitation.

The hypertensive disorders of pregnancy and their perpetuation of impaired renal perfusion are another important cause of AKI and generally occur in the later trimesters as well as the postpartum period. They include PEC with severe features, eclampsia, and HELLP (hemolysis, elevated liver enzymes and low platelet count) syndrome. In fact, AKI, including the presence of oliguria, is one of the parameters used to identify disease progression and disease recovery with its resolution. In general, profound AKI with oliguria occurs when both hypertensive disorders of pregnancy happen alongside hemorrhage, resulting in double and sustained insults to the renal system (3).

Finally, similar to the first trimester, severe infection can also cause renal impairment later in pregnancy or postpartum. The more common causes of sepsis at these later gestations include intrauterine inflammation or infection (Triple I) and pyelonephritis. Postpartum endometritis and postoperative complications, such as pelvic abscess or wound infection, are other common considerations.

Thrombotic thrombocytopenia purpura (TTP) and acute fatty liver of pregnancy (AFLP) are rare, but are severe causes of AKI in late pregnancy. Similarly, hemolytic uremic syndrome (HUS) is also a rare but a devastating cause of AKI that more commonly occurs postpartum (4). All three conditions share several features with PEC with HELLP syndrome, which can make it difficult to distinguish between them.

## Diagnostic Workup

The diagnostic workup for oliguria in a pregnant patient is relatively simple and should be guided by your clinical suspicions of the likely etiology. Following a careful history and physical exam, the use of further laboratory tests will be dictated by your differential. In all instances, the assessment of sCRT is helpful to better understand the extent of the AKI, keeping in mind the lower levels expected in pregnancy at baseline.

In clinical scenarios that remain unclear, one can use traditional strategies to distinguish between the various pathological causes of AKI (Table 9.3). This may include a detailed urinalysis with a microscopic

TABLE 9.3

Diagnostic Findings

| | |
|---|---|
| Prerenal (hypovolemia) | BUN/creatinine ratio > 20 |
| | • FeNa < 1% |
| | • Urine specific gravity > 1.018 |
| | • Hyaline casts in urinalysis |
| | • Improvement with IV fluid hydration |
| Intrinsic | Sepsis or ischemia |
| | • FeNa > 1% |
| | Hemolysis |
| | • Anemia |
| | • ↑ LDH |
| | • ↓ Haptogloblin |
| | TTP/HUS |
| | • Schistocytes on peripheral smear |
| | • ↑ LDH |
| | • Anemia |
| | • Thrombocytopenia |
| | Rhabdomyolysis |
| | • Urinalysis shows myoglobin, heme, limited red blood cells |
| | • ↑ Creatinine kinase |
| Postrenal | Obstruction |
| | • Hydronephrosis |
| | • Absent ureteral jets |

analysis that assesses not only for the presence of cells or protein, but also for the sedimentation and fractional excretion of sodium (FeNa). Additional tools include peripheral blood smears to assess for schistocytes or other signs of hemolysis.

When diagnosing PEC or distinguishing between HELLP, TTP/HUS, or AFLP, it is imperative to have a complete blood count, liver function tests, and lactate dehydrogenase (LDH) or haptoglobin.

In the setting of sepsis, lactic acid is an important marker of the extent of disease and a response to therapy. In addition, cultures of the urine, blood, and upper respiratory tract are crucial to identify an unknown source of infection and/or to isolate bacteria and their sensitivities.

In scenarios where postrenal obstruction is a concern, imaging with ultrasound for hydronephrosis or the identification of ureteral jets are useful tools. In some instances, computed tomography imaging is necessary for a more comprehensive diagnosis.

## Review of the Common Causes of Oliguria in Obstetrical Patients

### Preeclampsia with Severe Features or HELLP

PEC encompasses a spectrum of diseases, but can generally be thought of as a new onset of elevated blood pressures and proteinuria after 20 weeks of gestation. In its severe manifestations, renal insufficiency, inflammation of the liver, and neurological derangements are common features (6). HELLP syndrome is a variant of PEC and refers to a state of hemolysis, transaminitis, and thrombocytopenia. It can occur in the absence of HTN and proteinuria.

The pathophysiology of PEC is complex and not clearly understood. It is thought to be mediated by abnormal placentation, the release of pathological placental hormones, and endothelial leak. The latter not only causes the characteristic proteinuria of PEC, but also leads to the extravasation of fluid into the interstitium. This process compromises the normal physiological state of hypervolemia in pregnancy. The decrease in intravascular volume lowers preload, impairing cardiac output, and ultimately contributes to renal hypoperfusion. Furthermore, sustained elevations in blood pressure or afterload results in prolonged afferent arteriole vasoconstriction. The combination of the relative hypovolemia of PEC and the absence of compensatory afferent vasodilation leads to impaired GFR (7).

In addition, there are also subsequent morphological changes within the glomerular matrix, which involve the swelling or thickening of the glomerular endothelial cells, called endotheliosis (7). This results in the narrowing of the glomerular vessel lumens and its fenestrations, which impair filtration and leads to elevated sCRT levels. As the renal function continues to deteriorate, oliguria may develop. Some studies purport that oliguria may also be a reflection of acute deteriorations of renal function due to localized renal vasospasm (8).

Interestingly, the literature suggests that women who present with features of both severe PEC and HELLP are at the highest risk of oliguria and subsequent morbidity, such as requiring renal replacement therapy (7,9,10). Close attention to the renal function in these patients is paramount to preventing long-standing sequelae.

In the past, invasive hemodynamic monitoring with central venous catheters and pulmonary artery catheterizations were the mainstay in treating oliguria in the preeclamptic patient (8,9,11). The use of hydralazine, low-dose dopamine, and furosemide to improve the urine output was common, and their use was tailored toward the pathophysiology revealed through invasive monitoring (12–14). In most instances, oliguria was deemed to be a result of prerenal azotemia and resolved with adequate fluid resuscitation. However, localized renal vasospasm and persistently elevated systemic vascular resistance are two alternative processes described in the literature (8). For these specific instances, the use of vasodilators has been recommended to either locally target renal artery vasoconstriction or aggressively decrease afterload and preload, respectively.

However, these sophisticated titrations have since fallen out of favor in contemporary medical practices. There is now more focus on simply maintaining adequate blood pressure control, judicious intravenous fluid (IVF) hydration, avoidance of NSAIDs, the use of magnesium sulfate for seizure prophylaxis, and expeditious delivery when appropriate. Oliguria is expected to be resolved with these methods of stabilization (6,15–17). Of note, the use of magnesium sulfate in the setting of oliguria should be carefully done in order to prevent magnesium toxicity.

## Sepsis

Sepsis is a syndrome that results from the dysfunctional inflammatory response of the body to infection. Like PEC, it too represents a spectrum of diseases. Additionally, it too is one of the more common causes of AKI and oliguria in obstetric patients.

For example, the renal system is commonly affected by sepsis, which results in, elevated sCRT and oliguria.

A new screening tool for sepsis identification has been introduced called the quick Sepsis-related Organ Failure Assessment Score or qSOFA (18) (Table 9.4). It is primarily a tool for predicting poor prognosis for those patients with presumed sepsis and, as such, identifies those patients who may require higher levels of care. It is now the recommended tool for screening for severe sepsis in patients outside of the intensive care unit (ICU) setting.

The key in identifying sepsis is first suspecting an underlying infectious process. The source of infection will depend on the specifics of a patient's symptoms and clinical findings. The differential diagnosis of sepsis in obstetric patients can guide the clinician. It includes those infections that are common outside of pregnancy, such as pyelonephritis, pneumonia, influenza, appendicitis, or cholecystitis. Notably, these conditions, particularly pyelonephritis and influenza, are often more severe and exacerbated in the pregnant patient, requiring inpatient or even ICU-level care. Infections specific to obstetrics, include septic abortions, chorioamnionitis, endometritis, and postcesarean pelvic abscesses or wound infections.

Once sepsis is suspected, its treatment is universal regardless of pregnancy. The hallmark for treatment includes three major features: fluid resuscitation, antibiotic therapy, and source control (4). These are all markers for adequate resuscitation and/or need for more interventions such as vasopressors. In rare instances, renal AKI and subsequent oliguria are so extensive that renal replacement therapy with dialysis is necessary. This phenomenon is a relatively rare intervention needed for pregnant patients in the developed world (20).

Antibiotic therapy should target the microbiology most commonly associated with the presumed source. Finally, in many clinical scenarios, the removal of the cause of infection is key to successful treatment. For example, in some instances, uterine evacuation, via either delivery or dilation and curettage depending on antepartum or postpartum presentation, is necessary to obtain adequate source control.

An algorithm for oliguria management is shown in Figure 9.3.

TABLE 9.4

Quick Sepsis-Related Organ Failure Assessment Score[a]

| Two or more of the following: |
| --- |
| • Tachypnea > 21 minutes |
| • Systolic blood pressure < 101 mmHg |
| • Altered mental status (Glasgow Coma Scale < 15) |

[a] See further Singer et al. (18).

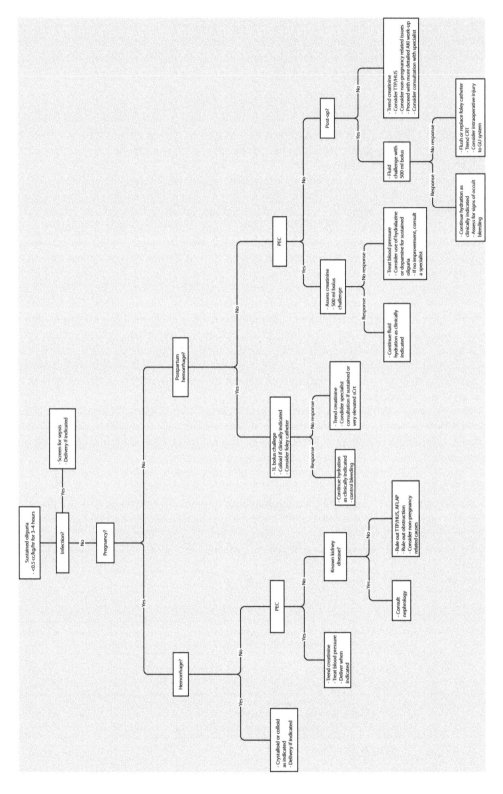

FIGURE 9.3 Oliguria management.

# REFERENCES

1. Kennedy BB, Harvey CJ, Saade GR. Acute renal failure. In: Troiano N, Harvey CJ, Chez BF, editors. *AWHONN high-risk and critical care obstetrics*. 3rd ed. Philadelphia, PA: Wolters Kluwer/Lippincott Williams & Wilkins; 2013.
2. Anantharaman P, Schmidt RJ, Holley JL. Pregnancy and renal disease. In: Lerma EV, Berns JS, Nissenson A, editors. *Current diagnosis and treatment: Nephrology and hypertension*. New York: McGraw-Hill Medical; 2009.
3. Renal and urinary tract disorders. In: Cunningham FG, Leveno KJ, Bloom SL, Spong CY, Dashe JS, Hoffman BL, Casey BM, Sheffield JS, editors. *Williams obstetrics*. 24th ed. New York: McGraw-Hill; 2013.
4. Robbins K, Martin S, Wilson W. Intensive care considerations for the critically ill parturient. In: Creasy R, Resnik R, Iams J, Lockwood C, Moore T, Greene M, editors. *Creasy and Resnik's maternal-fetal medicine: Principles and practice*. 7th ed. Philadelphia, PA: Elsevier; 2014; 1182-1214.
5. Waikar SS, Bonventre JV. Acute kidney injury. In: Kasper D, Hauser SL, Jameson JL, Fauci AS, Longo DL, Loscalzo J, editors. *Harrison's principles of internal medicine*. 19th ed. New York: McGraw-Hill Medical; 2015.
6. Roberts JM, August PA, Bakris G, Barton JR, Bernstein, IM, Druzin, M et al. ACOG guidelines: Hypertension in pregnancy. *Obs Gynecol*. 2013; 122(5):1122-1131.
7. Hypertensive disorders. In: Cunningham F, Leveno KJ, Bloom SL, Spong CY, Dashe JS, Hoffman BL, Casey BM, Sheffield JS, editors. *Williams obstetrics*. 24th ed. New York: McGraw-Hill; 2013. Available from http://accessmedicine.mhmedical.com/content.aspx?bookid=1057&sectionid=59789184 [Accessed November 12, 2017].
8. Clark SL, Greenspoon JS, Aldahl D, Phelan JP. Severe preeclampsia with persistent oliguria: Management of hemodynamic subsets. *Am J Obstet Gynecol*. 1986; 154(3):490-494.
9. Markham K, Funai E. Pregnany-related hypertension. In: Creasy R, Resnik R, Iams J, Lockwood C, Moore T, Greene M, editors. *Creasy and Resnik's maternal-fetal medicine: Principles and practice*. 7th ed. Philadelphia, PA: Elsevier; 2014; 756-784.
10. Silva GB Jr, Monteiro FA, Mota RM, Paiva JG, Correia JW, Bezerra Filho JG et al. Acute kidney injury requiring dialysis in obstetric patients: A series of 55 cases in Brazil. *Arch Gynecol Obstet*. 2009; 279(2):131-137.
11. Clark SL, Hankins GD. Preventing maternal death: 10 clinical diamonds. *Obs Gynecol*. 2012; 119:360–364.
12. Katz VL, Dotters DJ, Droegemueller W. Low dose dopamine in the treatment of persistent oliguria in pre-eclampsia. *Int J Gynecol Obstet*. 1990; 31(1):57-59.
13. Keiseb J, Moodley J, Connolly CA. Comparison of the efficacy of continuous furosemide and low-dose dopamine infusion in pre-eclampsia/eclampsia related oliguria in the immediate postpartum period. *Hypertens Pregnancy*. 2002; 21(3):225-234.
14. Mantel GD, Makin JD. Low dose dopamine in postpartum pre-eclamptic women with oliguria: A double-blind, placebo controlled, randomised trial. *Br J Obstet Gynaecol*. 1997; 104(11):80-81.
15. Rose B, Spencer R, Hensleigh P. Resolution of oliguria in a pre-eclamptic after treatment with magnesium sulfate. *J Perinatol*. 1987; VII(3):215-216.
16. Mantel GD. Care of the critically ill parturient: Oliguria and renal failure. *Best Pract Res Clin Obstet Gynaecol*. 2001; 15(4):563-581.
17. Alexander JM, Wilson KL. Hypertensive emergencies of pregnancy. *Obstet Gynecol Clin North Am*. 2013; 40(1):89-101.
18. Singer M, Deutschman CS, Seymour CW, Shankar-Hari M, Annane D, Bauer M et al. The third international consensus definitions for sepsis and septic shock (Sepsis-3). *JAMA*. 2016; 315(8):801-810.
19. Bauer ME, Bauer ST, Rajala B, MacEachern MP, Polley LS, Childers D et al. Maternal physiologic parameters in relationship to systemic inflammatory response syndrome criteria: A systematic review and meta-analysis. *Obstet Gynecol*. 2014; 124(3):535-541.
20. Ali A, Ali MA, Ali MU, Mohammad S. Hospital outcomes of obstetrical-related acute renal failure in a tertiary care teaching. *Ren Fail*. 2011; 33(3):285-290.

# 10

## Seizures

**Neil S. Seligman, MD**

### CONTENTS

## Introduction

Acute seizures are a common medical emergency which can result in serious physical trauma or death. Even one seizure can have major social and emotional consequences such as the loss of driving privileges, limitations for employment, loss of independence, and damage to self-esteem (1). Approximately 10% of the population of the United States will suffer a seizure at some point in their lifetime and approximately 2% will develop epilepsy (2). The annual incidence of seizures ranges from 70 to 100 per 100,000 population (3). Acute seizures result in 1,000,000 emergency room visits accounting for 1% of emergency room visits overall (4).

Pregnant women are particularly likely to seek care in the emergency room or on labor and delivery following a seizure. Seizures can harm not only the woman but also the fetus as a result of injury from falls and/or hypoxia, which, if sustained, can lead to acidosis and fetal death (5). Convulsions may also cause electrolyte abnormalities, changes in blood pressure, and alterations in uterine blood flow (6). Frequent seizures may adversely affect fetal neurodevelopment (7). Maternal death may result from accidental death, sudden unexpected death in epilepsy, death from status epilepticus (SE), suicide, and medication complications (e.g., toxicity) (7). The overall incidence of seizures during pregnancy is not well defined; however, epilepsy is one of the most common medical conditions in reproductive-age women, affecting an estimated 1.1 million women overall and 0.3–0.6% of pregnant women (8,9).

## Etiology

Seizures may be provoked or unprovoked. A *provoked* seizure is an epileptic seizure caused by an acute medical or neurological illness or injury (e.g., hypoglycemia), whereas an *unprovoked* seizure is a seizure of unknown etiology or a seizure due to a preexisting brain lesion or progressive central nervous system (CNS) disorder (10). In a study which included 564 patients with definite epileptic seizure, 62% were idiopathic. In the remainder, acute or remote symptomatic seizures, vascular disease, and tumors were the most common causes (11). Other important terminologies are defined in Table 10.1.

Epilepsy and eclampsia are the most common causes of seizures during pregnancy (12,13). Epilepsy may appear for the first time during (referred to as gestational-onset epilepsy) or shortly after pregnancy (9). Among women with epilepsy, 12.8% report onset during pregnancy, which is either due to coincidence or the activation of a seizure focus as a result of the physiological changes that occur in

**TABLE 10.1**

Terminology

---

- Epileptic seizures
  - Temporary alteration in behavior resulting from a sudden, abnormal burst of electrical activity in the brain
- Non-epileptic seizures
  - Mimics epileptic seizure without the neurophysiological changes associated with an epileptic seizure
- Focal seizures
  - Replaces the term *partial seizure*; originate in one hemisphere of the brain
  - Symptoms depend on where the seizure originates in the brain and can include motor, somatosensory, sensory, autonomic, or psychic symptoms
  - Simple (normal awareness) or complex (impaired awareness)
- Generalized seizures
  - Originate in both hemispheres of the brain; may be convulsive or nonconvulsive
  - Tonic–clonic; abrupt, generalized, bilateral muscle stiffening and subsequent rhythmic jerking of the limbs; other common features include tongue biting, incontinence, and impaired consciousness
  - Absence; also called petit mal seizures; brief staring episodes with impaired consciousness; may be atypical (changes in tone and cessation are not abrupt) and/or accompanied by myoclonia
  - Clonic (rhythmic jerking muscle contractions), myoclonic (brief muscle contractions usually without impaired consciousness), tonic (sudden muscle stiffening often with impaired consciousness and falling), atonic (aka drop seizures; sudden loss of muscle control)
- Unknown seizures
  - Seizures which cannot be classified as focal or generalized
- Generalized convulsive status epilepticus
  - A single epileptic seizure of >30 minutes in duration or a series of seizures over 30 minutes between which normal function is not regained
- Nonconvulsive status epilepticus
  - Ongoing or intermittent seizure activity without convulsions for at least 5–10 minutes, without recovery of consciousness between attacks or >50% ictal EEG activity over a 60-minute period in patients with baseline coma or encephalopathy

---

pregnancy (14). Gestational epilepsy is a rare condition characterized by seizures occurring only during pregnancy. In the acute setting, gestational epilepsy may be indistinguishable from gestational-onset epilepsy. Importantly, a history of epilepsy should not be the rationale for failing to perform a thorough evaluation for other causes of seizure, especially when the seizure is different from the patient's past seizures (new focal component or neurological deficit; Table 10.2). Among women with epilepsy, 14–32% will experience an increase in the frequency of seizures during pregnancy (9) due to the following:

- Poor-compliance antiepileptic drugs (AEDs)
- Changes in AED levels from altered metabolism, decreased protein binding, increased clearance, impaired absorption, and increased volume of distribution (12)
- Dehydration
- Sleep deprivation
- Use of analgesics (e.g., meperidine), which lower seizure threshold (8,12)

Eclampsia is the most common cause of new-onset seizures during pregnancy (12) and can result in significant maternal (e.g., intracerebral hemorrhage, liver hematoma) and fetal (e.g., abruption, stillbirth) morbidity. In developed countries, the risk of death is low (<1%). Eclampsia occurs in 2–3% of women with preeclampsia (PEC) with severe features and 0.6% of women with PEC without severe features (15). Without magnesium, 10% of eclamptic women will have a repeat seizure (16). The most common preceding symptoms are visual changes, headaches, and/or epigastric pain. Proteinuria or hypertension are absent in 38% of women at the time of the seizure (12,17). Eclampsia can occur before or after delivery (44%), usually within the first 48 hours (17); postpartum eclampsia carries a worse prognosis because of a more frequent association with adult respiratory distress syndrome and disseminated intravascular coagulation (12).

TABLE 10.2

Common Causes of Epileptic Seizure and Common Characteristics

- Epilepsy
- Hypoglycemia
  - More common in diabetics taking insulin and oral hypoglycemic drugs
  - Islet cell tumors
  - Preceded by diaphoresis, tachycardia, anxiety, and confusion
- Nonketotic hyperglycemia
  - More common in the elderly; causes focal motor seizures
- Eclampsia
- Acute hepatitis
  - Acute fatty liver of pregnancy
  - Viral hepatitis
- Electrolyte abnormalities
  - Hyponatremia; seizure often preceded by confusion and altered consciousness
  - Hypocalcemia associated with thyroid or parathyroid surgery, renal failure, hypoparathyroidism, and pancreatitis; seizure often preceded by mental status changes and tetany
  - Hypomagnesemia; seizure often preceded by irritability, agitation, confusion, myoclonus, tetany, and convulsions; may be accompanied by hypocalcemia
- Inborn error of metabolism
- Hypoxia and cerebral anoxia
  - CO poisoning
  - Cardiac and respiratory arrest
  - Complications of anesthesia
- Medication toxicity
  - E.g., isoniazid, heterocyclic antidepressants, cyanide
- Conditions affecting the CNS
  - Head trauma
  - Brain tumor
  - Cerebrovascular disease (e.g., stroke)
  - Intracranial or subarachnoid hemorrhage
  - Infection (e.g., encephalitis)
  - Congenital malformation
    - Cerebral venous sinus thrombosis; seizure present in 50%. Symptoms also include headache (95%), papilledema, and/or altered mental status (~33%).
  - Posterior reversible encephalopathy syndrome or reversible cerebral vasoconstriction syndrome
- Alcohol or drug withdrawal
  - Typically 7–48 hours after the last drink
- Drug intoxication
- Renal failure and uremia
  - Associated with myoclonic and generalized tonic–clonic seizures
- Hyperthyroidism
- Rare
  - Thrombotic thrombocytopenic purpura
  - Cerebral lupus
  - Dialysis disequilibrium syndrome
  - Porphyria
    - Preceded by abdominal pain and behavioral changes; diagnosed by urine porphyrin and porphobilinogen
  - Malaria

Intracranial hemorrhage and subarachnoid hemorrhage are responsible for only a small proportion of seizures in pregnant women but mortality ranges from 40% to 75% (12,18,19); because of the critical nature of these conditions, new-onset seizures during pregnancy should be assumed to be due to eclampsia, intracranial hemorrhage, or subarachnoid hemorrhage until proven otherwise (20). Seizures with a focal component in particular require careful evaluation. Other causes of "seizure-like" activity are shown in Table 10.3.

TABLE 10.3

Differential Diagnosis and Differentiating Characteristics

- Complex migraine (presents with headache)
  - Syncope (brief—few seconds to 1 minute and no postictal confusion)
- Psychological disorders (e.g., hallucinations)
- Psychogenic nonepileptic seizure
- Transient ischemic attack or other neurological events (may mimic a focal seizure)
- Tremor, paroxysmal movement disorders
- Medication-induced dystonia (e.g., haloperidol, promethazine, metoclopramide)
- Sleep disorders (e.g., narcolepsy; patients feel refreshed after episode)
- Sleep starts (sudden, brief, strong contractions of the body or parts of the body that occur while falling asleep)

## Initial Management

The initial management of an actively seizing pregnant woman is shown in Figures 10.1 and 10.2. Management is similar to that of the nonpregnant patient with a few additional considerations. Tongue biting is common with generalized tonic–clonic seizures; however, nothing should be placed in the mouth. An oral airway may be needed to protect the patency of the airway but placement can be challenging in an actively seizing patient. Most seizures will resolve within 2–3 minutes regardless of intervention. No drugs used in the emergency management of seizures should be withheld due to concerns for fetal risk. Benzodiazepines are considered the first-line medication for acute seizures and are safe during pregnancy. A recent meta-analysis of first-trimester exposure to benzodiazepines did not demonstrate an increase in major malformations (odds ratio: 1.06; 95% confidence interval: 0.91–1.25) (21,22); neonatal withdrawal is unlikely with intermittent use as in the acute management of seizures. Phenytoin and phenobarbital can also be safely used. Suggested doses are shown in Figure 10.2.

SE, which complicates 1–2% of pregnancies (12), is associated with significant maternal and fetal morbidity and mortality without aggressive treatment. In the general population, mortality ranges from 6 to 28% (23,24). Morbidities include the following:

- Refractory seizures (25%)
- Epilepsy (41%)
- Deterioration in function (25%)
- Need for long-term care (10%)
- Chronic encephalopathy (10%) (25)

In a report of SE in pregnancy among 29 cases of SE, there were 9 maternal deaths (31%) and 14 infant deaths (48%) (5). However, in a more recent study of 3806 pregnancies of women with epilepsy, there were no maternal mortalities, no miscarriages, and only a single stillbirth among 21 cases of SE with standardized treatment (26).

The early treatment of SE is essential since the risk of seizures becoming self-sustaining begins to increase after as little as 10 minutes. To avoid morbidity and the development of refractory seizures, a reasonable operational definition of SE is "a seizure lasting 5 minutes or more or 2 or more seizures between which there is incomplete recovery of consciousness" (25). In practice, the treatment of generalized convulsive SE should be initiated for any woman with a seizure that does not self-terminate or respond to initial treatment (27) with the input of an experienced team of neurologists and critical care specialists. Delivery should be considered if the fetus is viable.

If feasible, fetal heart monitoring and tocometry can be initiated during a seizure if the fetus has a gestational age of >23 weeks, but temporary fetal heart rate changes should be anticipated. Fetal bradycardia for at least 3–5 minutes is common during and after an eclamptic seizure (28,29). Fetal tachycardia, loss of heart rate variability, and sometimes transient decelerations may persist for some time after the resolution of the seizure. When these heart rate abnormalities are seen, the main focus should remain

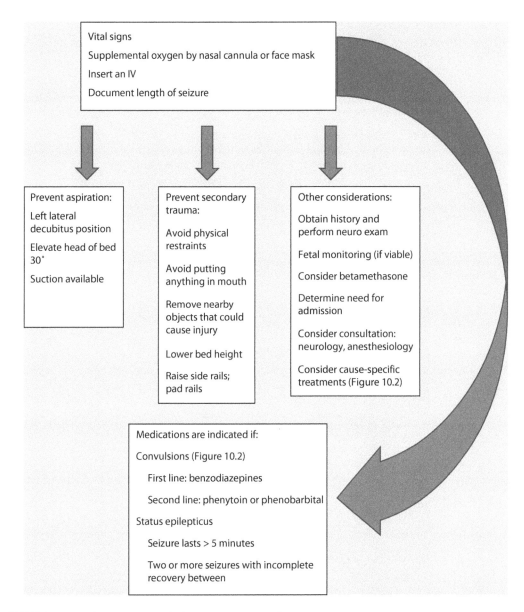

Vital signs

Supplemental oxygen by nasal cannula or face mask

Insert an IV

Document length of seizure

Prevent aspiration:

Left lateral decubitus position

Elevate head of bed 30°

Suction available

Prevent secondary trauma:

Avoid physical restraints

Avoid putting anything in mouth

Remove nearby objects that could cause injury

Lower bed height

Raise side rails; pad rails

Other considerations:

Obtain history and perform neuro exam

Fetal monitoring (if viable)

Consider betamethasone

Determine need for admission

Consider consultation: neurology, anesthesiology

Consider cause-specific treatments (Figure 10.2)

Medications are indicated if:

Convulsions (Figure 10.2)

First line: benzodiazepines

Second line: phenytoin or phenobarbital

Status epilepticus

Seizure lasts > 5 minutes

Two or more seizures with incomplete recovery between

FIGURE 10.1    Initial management of seizure in a pregnant patient.

the treatment of the seizure; delivery during or immediately following a seizure should be avoided in the absence of fetal heart changes suggestive of impending fetal injury or death. If abdominal trauma occurred during the seizure, at least 4 hours of continuous fetal monitoring is suggested.

After the seizure is resolved, management should focus on the evaluation (Figure 10.3) and, if appropriate, treatment of the underlying cause. An accurate history is important. Among individuals with supposedly new-onset seizures, studies show that 50% of these individuals, with careful history taking, actually have had a prior seizure and warrant a diagnosis of epilepsy (30). In addition to the typical elements of a history, the history should also include the following details:

- A description of the seizure
- Recollection of events immediately preceding, during, or after the seizure
- Aura or prodromal symptoms

**Medication doses**

- First line: benzodiazepines
  - Lorazepam 2–4 mg IV over 2–3 min, repeat in 10–15 min ×1; may give IM
  - Diazepam 5–10 mg IV over 1–2 min q 5–10 min, max 30 mg; may give IM or PR (gel)
  - Midazolam (Versed) 1–2 mg IV q 5 min, max 10 mg
- Second line: phenytoin or phenobarbital
  - Phenytoin 15–20 mg/kg IV, repeat 10 mg/kg after 20 min; avoid with hypotension. Continue until 24 hours after extubated and/or returned to baseline MS
  - Phenobarbital 100 mg/min until seizure stops or max 20 mg/kg

**Cause specific treatment considerations**

- Eclampsia → Magnesium load 10 gm IM or 4 gm IV, antihypertensive medications, delivery
- Hypoglycemia → 50% dextrose 50 ml IV
- Alcohol → Thiamine 100 mg IM or IV prior to glucose
- Drug toxicity/poisoning → Give antidote if available

FIGURE 10.2   Treatment options.

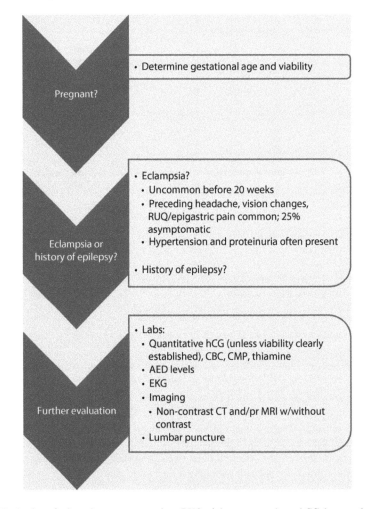

FIGURE 10.3   Evaluation of seizure in a pregnant patient. RUQ, right upper quadrant; hCG, human chorionic gonadotropin; CBC, complete blood count; CMP, complete metabolic panel.

- Postictal symptoms
- Recent sleep deprivation
- History of head trauma, meningitis, vascular disease, or stroke
- Medication history
- Recent medication changes (e.g., discontinuation of benzodiazepines or barbiturates)
- AED use
- Any potential precipitant or trigger
- History of previous seizures and family history of seizures
- History of alcoholism

Physical examination should include a thorough neurological exam with the assessment of the following:

- Cranial nerves
- Orientation
- Motor strength
- Sensory perception
- Reflexes

Lateralizing signs may indicate a contralateral structural brain lesion.

The diagnostic evaluation focuses on identifying dangerous and reversible causes. Electroencephalogram (EEG) and brain imaging (to rule out structural lesions) should be considered a routine part of the evaluation of an adult presenting with an apparent unprovoked first seizure (31). The EEG will reveal epileptiform abnormalities in 23–29% of patients. These findings may be helpful in diagnosing and classifying the seizure, predicting seizure recurrence, and guiding treatment (24,31). A normal EEG (approximately 30% of individuals) does not exclude the presence of a seizure disorder (32).

Brain imaging (computed tomography [CT] or magnetic resonance imaging [MRI] scans) has a yield of about 10% (31). Positive findings are more likely if the neurological exam is abnormal. Abnormalities which may affect management include previously unrecognized brain tumors, vascular lesions, and cerebral cysticercosis (31). An emergent noncontrast head CT scan is recommended in patients with a history or findings of trauma, history of malignancy, immunocompromised state, fever, persistent headaches, history of anticoagulation, or history of new focal neurological deficits or focal onset of seizures with or without generalization (33). Exposure to <50 mGy has not been associated with an increased risk of fetal anomalies, pregnancy loss, or adverse neurodevelopmental outcome (34). Fetal exposure to more than 10–20 mGy of ionizing radiation is associated with a 1.5–2.0 times increased risk of childhood leukemia; however, the attributable risk is small (1 additional case per 6000 children). Diagnostic imaging with ionizing radiation should not be withheld solely due to concern for fetal exposure. Typical fetal exposure from a head CT scan is <0.5 mGy and can be minimized with the use of appropriate shielding. MRI with or without contrast is more sensitive and is preferred in the nonemergent setting. Outpatient imaging may be reasonable in a patient who has returned to baseline and has a normal neurological exam, and reliable follow-up can be arranged (27,35). Gadolinium crosses the placenta and is typically avoided during pregnancy because of lack of safety data, although no adverse effects have been reported.

Additional evaluation may include lumbar puncture, blood work, and urine toxicology, but there is insufficient evidence to recommend these tests routinely (30,31). Lumbar puncture may be helpful in specific situations, such as when the presentation includes fever or in an immunocompromised patient (27,35). An abnormal white blood cell count is not uncommon (29% of new-onset seizures and 4% of recurrent seizures) but rarely alters management (36). In general, the yield of blood work is lower in patients whose symptoms have resolved. Normal physiological changes in laboratory values that occur during pregnancy should be considered when in interpreting blood work results. Seizures have been reported due to intoxication with selective serotonin reuptake inhibitors, cocaine, and other stimulants;

toxicology rarely alters management but has implications for neonatal care and management. Alcohol-related and alcohol withdrawal seizures are a diagnosis of exclusion.

---

## After Initial Management

The postictal state is a period of transition back to normal awareness and function lasting several minutes to hours or even days. Confusion, decreased alertness, and focal neurological deficits are typical and should gradually improve. Weakness, called postictal paresis or Todd's paralysis, is present in approximately 13.4% of patients and may last hours to days (37). Other postictal symptoms may include transient aphasia, amaurosis, hemi anopsia, sensory loss, psychosis, and aggression. Hospitalization is not necessary if the neurological exam is normal and mental status has returned to baseline. Nonetheless, admission is common in pregnant women with new-onset seizures.

The recurrence risk is highest in the first 2 years after a seizure. Rates of recurrence are 10% in the first year and 24% (range 21–45%) by 2 years (1). Considering only patients with an unprovoked first seizure, 40–52% will have a second seizure and 60–90% will have additional seizures by 4 years (38,39). Characteristics which impart the highest risk of recurrence are prior brain insult or brain lesion (hazard ratio [HR] 2.55; 1.44–4.51), significant brain imaging abnormalities (HR 2.44 1.09–5.44), nocturnal seizures (HR 2.1; 1.0–4.3), and/or epileptiform activity on EEG (HR 2.16 1.07–4.38) (1). Other factors, including multiple seizures within 24 hours, were not related to the risk of recurrence. Women are no more likely than men to have a recurrent seizure.

The decision to start AEDs is based on several factors including recurrence risk and adverse effect profile. AED treatment is rarely started after a first unprovoked seizure. Immediate AED therapy (within 3 months after the seizure) reduces the risk of seizure recurrence in the subsequent 2 years by 35% (range: 23–46%) but is unlikely to improve prognosis for long-term sustained seizure remission and quality of life or to reduce the risk of sudden death (1). Therefore, patients at the lowest risk of recurrence, including those with a normal neurological exam, no comorbidities, no known structural brain disease, and/or seizure due to a secondary cause, do not need to start AEDs. On the other hand, for patients who have a second seizure, the risk of recurrence is 57% in the first year and 73% by 4 years; AEDs should be started in these patients (1). Other patients who are at a high risk of recurrence include patients with a structural brain lesion (recurrence of up to 65%), history of brain injury, family history of seizures, spike and wave pattern on EEG, and postictal paresis. Short-term AEDs should also be considered when a transient risk factor remains present (e.g., ongoing metabolic abnormality). Furthermore, any circumstance where the risk of recurrence approaches that of a patient for whom immediate treatment would generally be considered should start AEDs.

Monotherapy improves tolerability and compliance and reduces adverse events (AEs) and drug interactions. AEs range from 7% to 31%, although most are mild and reversible (1). Most AEs are dose related and improve with dose reduction or discontinuation. The choice of AED should be based, at least in part, on seizure type, comorbidities, and pregnancy risk. Actual teratogenic risk is very low with most AEDs. Regardless, the risk of congenital anomalies is limited to a very small window during fetal development. Organ formation begins in the embryonic period (second week after conception or fourth week after the first day of the last menstrual period) and is complete by the early part of the fetal period (typically 10 weeks after conception or 12 weeks after the first day of the last menstrual period). Before this time, if damage were to occur due to medication exposure, the result would be a miscarriage, whereas later exposure may result in developmental defects. An example of this is valproate. Valproate use during pregnancy is associated with not only major congenital malformations, but also lower intelligence quotient, poorer performance on tests of mental and motor ability, and an increased risk of autism spectrum disorders when used in the second and third trimesters; for these reasons, valproate is typically avoided unless absolutely necessary (e.g., preexisting epilepsy refractory to multiple other medications). The decision to start treatment with an AED, and the choice of AED, is typically made in concert with a neurologist. Lamotrigine may be a good first choice based on the availability of safety data but needs to be slowly titrated because it has the potential to cause the Stevens–Johnson syndrome. Dosing should be the lowest dose that controls breakthrough seizures. After discharge home and regardless of whether medications are started, the patient should have a follow-up with their obstetrician and a neurologist. The need for specific precautions varies from patient to patient. Most states require a specific seizure-free period before allowing patients to drive, but other factors such as medication effects (e.g., blurry vision) should be considered. The ability to return to work and participation in sports require careful assessment by a neurologist familiar with these issues.

## REFERENCES

1. Krumholz A, Wiebe S, Gronseth GS, Gloss DS, Sanchez AM, Kabir AA et al. Evidence-based guideline: Management of an unprovoked first seizure in adults: Report of the Guideline Development Subcommittee of the American Academy of Neurology and the American Epilepsy Society. *Neurology*. 2015 Apr; 84(16):1705-1713.
2. Middleton DB. Seizures. In: South-Paul JE, Matheny SC, Lewis EL, editors. *CURRENT diagnosis & treatment: Family medicine*. 4th ed. New York: McGraw-Hill; 2015. Available from: http://accessmedicine.mhmedical.com/content.aspx?bookid=1415&sectionid=77054981.
3. Hauser WA, Beghi E. First seizure definitions and worldwide incidence and mortality. *Epilepsia*. 2008 Jan; 49(s1):8-12.
4. Pallin DJ, Goldstein JN, Moussally JS, Pelletier AJ, Green AR, Camargo, Jr. CA. Seizure visits in US emergency departments: Epidemiology and potential disparities in care. *Int J Emerg Med*. 2008 Jun; 1(2):97-105.
5. Teramo K, Hiilesmaa V. Pregnancy and fetal complications in epileptic pregnancies: Review of the literature. In: Janz D, Dam M, Richens A et al., editors. *Epilepsy, pregnancy and the child*. New York: Raven Press; 1982, pp. 53-58.
6. Barrett C, Richens A. Epilepsy and pregnancy: Report of an Epilepsy Research Foundation Workshop. *Epilepsy Res*. 2003 Jan; 52(3):147-187.
7. Harini C, Mnatsakanyan L. New onset seizures during pregnancy. In: Sazgar M, Harden CL, editors. *Controversies in caring for women with epilepsy*. Cham: Springer International; 2016, pp. 107-113.
8. Epilepsy Foundation. *Risks during pregnancy* [Internet]. Landover, MD: Epilepsy Foundation. Available from: http://www.epilepsy.com/learn/impact/reproductive-risks/risks-during-pregnancy [Accessed August 28, 2016].
9. Aminoff MJ, Douglas VC. Neurologic disorders. In: Creasy RK, Resnik R, Iams JD et al., editors. *Maternal-fetal medicine: Principles and practice*. 7th ed. Philadelphia, PA: Elsevier; 2014, pp. 1100-1121.
10. Karceski S. Initial treatment of epilepsy in adults. In: Pedley TA, editor. *UpToDate*. Waltham, MA: UpToDate; 2016.
11. Sander JW, Hart YM, Shorvon SD, Johnson AL. Medical science: National general practice study of epilepsy: Newly diagnosed epileptic seizures in a general population. *Lancet*. 1990 Nov; 336(8726):1267-1271.
12. Beach RL, Kaplan PW. Seizures in pregnancy: Diagnosis and management. *Int Rev Neurobiol*. 2008 Dec; 83:259-271.
13. Wilson KL, Alexander JM. Seizures and intracranial hemorrhage. *Obstet Gynecol Clin North Am*. 2013 Mar; 40(1):103-120.
14. Jagoda A, Riggio S. Emergency department approach to managing seizures in pregnancy. *Ann Emerg Med*. 1991 Jan; 20(1):80-85.
15. Sibai BM. Magnesium sulfate prophylaxis in preeclampsia: Lessons learned from recent trials. *Am J Obstet Gynecol*. 2004 Jun; 190(6):1520-1526.
16. Pritchard JA, Cunningham FG, Pritchard SA. The Parkland Memorial Hospital protocol for treatment of eclampsia: Evaluation of 245 cases. *Am J Obstet Gynecol*. 1984 Apr; 148(7):951-963.
17. Roberts JM, Redman CW. Pre-eclampsia: More than pregnancy-induced hypertension. *Lancet*. 1993 Jun; 341(8858):1447-1451.
18. Munnur U, Karnad DR, Bandi VD, Lapsia V, Suresh MS et al. Critically ill obstetric patients in an American and an Indian public hospital: Comparison of case-mix, organ dysfunction, intensive care requirements, and outcomes. *Intensive Care Med*. 2005 Aug; 31(8):1087-1094.
19. Shehata HA, Okosun H. Neurological disorders in pregnancy. *Curr Opin Obstet Gynecol*. 2004 Apr; 16(2):117-122.

20. Guntupalli KK, Karnad DR, Bandi V, Hall N, Belfort M. Critical illness in pregnancy: Part II: Common medical conditions complicating pregnancy and puerperium. *CHEST J.* 2015 Nov; 148(5):1333-1345.

21. Organization of Teratology Information Specialists. *Benzodiazepines and pregnancy.* Reston, VA: Organization of Teratology Information Specialists. Available from: http://mothertobaby.org/fact-sheets /benzodiazepines-pregnancy [Accessed August 28, 2016].

22. Enato E, Moretti M, Koren G. Motherisk rounds: The fetal safety of benzodiazepines: An updated meta-analysis. *J Obstet Gynaecol Cana.* 2011 Jan; 33(1):46-48.

23. Celesia GG. Modern concepts of status epilepticus. *JAMA.* 1976 Apr; 235(15):1571-1574.

24. Bhanushali MJ, Helmers SJ. Diagnosis and acute management of seizure in adults. *Hosp Physician.* 2008 Nov;48:37-42.

25. Foreman B, Hirsch LJ. Epilepsy emergencies: Diagnosis and management. *Neurol Clin.* 2012 Feb; 30(1):11-41.

26. Battino D, Tomson T, Bonizzoni E, Craig J, Lindhout D, Sabers A et al. Seizure control and treatment changes in pregnancy: Observations from the EURAP epilepsy pregnancy registry. *Epilepsia.* 2013 Sep; 54(9):1621-1627.

27. EB Medicine. *Current guidelines for management of seizures in the emergency department.* Williamsport, PA: EB Medicine. Available from: http://www.ebmedicine.net/topics.php?paction=showTopic&topic _id=212 [Accessed August 28, 2016].

28. Norwitz ER. Eclampsia. In: Lockwood CJ, Pedley TA, editors. *UpToDate.* Waltham, MA: UpToDate; 2016.

29. Paul RH, Koh KS, Bernstein SG. Changes in fetal heart rate-uterine contraction patterns associated with eclampsia. *Am J Obstet Gynecol.* 1978 Jan; 130(2):165-169.

30. Krumholz A, Wiebe S, Gronseth G, Shinnar S, Levisohn P, Ting T et al. Practice parameter: Evaluating an apparent unprovoked first seizure in adults (an evidence-based review): Report of the Quality Standards Subcommittee of the American Academy of Neurology and the American Epilepsy Society. *Neurology.* 2007 Nov; 69(21):1996-2007.

31. American Academy of Neurology. *Evaluating an apparent unprovoked first seizure in adults.* Minneapolis, MN: American Academy of Neurology. Available from: https://www.aan.com/Guidelines /home/GetGuidelineContent/271 [Accessed August 28, 2016].

32. Schreiner A, Pohlmann-Eden B. Value of the early electroencephalogram after a first unprovoked seizure. *Clin EEG Neurosci.* 2003 Jul; 34(3):140-144.

33. American College of Emergency Physicians, American Academy of Neurology, American Association of Neurological Surgeons, American Society of Neuroradiology. Practice parameter: Neuroimaging in the emergency patient presenting with seizure (summary statement). *Ann Emerg Med.* 1996 Jul; 28(1):114-118.

34. ACOG Committee on Obstetric Practice. ACOG Committee Opinion. Number 299, September 2004 (replaces No. 158, September 1995). Guidelines for diagnostic imaging during pregnancy. *Obstet Gynecol.* 2004 Sep; 104(3):647-651.

35. Huff JS, Melnick ER, Tomaszewski CA, Theissen ME, Jagoda AS, Fesmire FM et al. Clinical policy: Critical issues in the evaluation and management of adult patients presenting to the emergency department with seizures. *Ann Emerg Med.* 2014 Apr; 63(4):437-447.

36. Bradford JC, Kyriakedes CG. Evaluation of the patient with seizures: An evidence based approach. *Emerg Med Clin North Am.* 1999 Feb; 17(1):203-220.

37. Gallmetzer P, Leutmezer F, Serles W, Assem-Hilger E, Spatt J, Baumgartner C. Postictal paresis in focal epilepsies—Incidence, duration, and causes: A video-EEG monitoring study. *Neurology.* 2004 Jun; 62(12):2160-2164.

38. Hauser WA, Hesdorffer DC *Epilepsy: Frequency, causes and consequences.* New York: Demos Medical Publishing; 1990.

39. Fisher RS, Acevedo C, Arzimanoglou A, Bogacz A, Cross JH, Elger CE et al. ILAE Official Report: A practical clinical definition of epilepsy. *Epilepsia.* 2014 April; 55(4):475-482.

# 11

## Acute Mental Status Change

Matthew K. Hoffman, MD, MPH, FACOG and Victoria Greenberg, MD

CONTENTS

## Initial Assessment

The initial approach to the pregnant patient with AMS begins with a primary survey with the goal of first stabilizing the mother and then addressing the fetus. The ABCs (airway, breathing, and circulation) of advanced cardiac life support need to be immediately implemented and adapted to the pregnant patient, particularly deviating the uterus off the vena cava (Figure 11.1) (1,2).

Assuming that the patient does not require acute resuscitation, the provider must move beyond the ABCs and assess the following:

- *D—Disability level*: The patient's disability level can be typically assessed by using the Glasgow Coma Scale or the AVPU scale (Figure 11.2) (the patient's *a*lertness, response to *v*oice, localization to *p*ain stimuli, or *u*nresponsive should be noted).
- *E—Exposure*: The last step in the primary survey is a rapid head-to-toe examination after fully undressing the patient. Observe for signs of trauma, medication patches, catheters, rashes, track marks, or wounds that can provide information about the etiology of the patient's mental status.
- *F—Fetus*: Fetal monitoring should begin *as soon as* a decision has been made that the fetus is viable and delivery does not unnecessarily compromise the mother's health or a perimortem section is indicated.

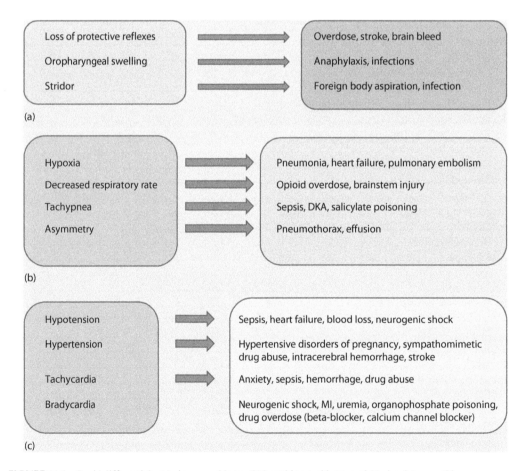

FIGURE 11.1   Rapid differentials: (a) airway problems, (b) breathing problems, and (c) circulatory problems.

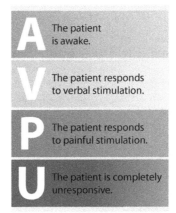

FIGURE 11.2   AVPU scale.

In order to improve both neonatal and maternal survival in a perimortem cesarean delivery, the delivery should begin 4 minutes after cardiac arrest. In addition to the neonatal benefits, delivery allows improvement in maternal cardiopulmonary resuscitation due to improved venous return and an increase in cardiac output to the rest of the body.

## Rapid Interventions

Following the initial assessment, the focus shifts to rapid interventions to identify and treat fixable causes of AMS. Blood glucose should be measured. If hypoglycemia is found, the patient should immediately be given an ampule of D50 or juice if intravenous (IV) access is unavailable. If narcotic overdose is suspected, 1–2 mg IV naloxone should be administered. If the patient has a history of alcoholism, hyperemesis gravidarum, or eating disorder or is on total parenteral nutrition, administer 100 mg IV thiamine before giving dextrose-containing IV fluid. After stabilizing the patient and correcting rapidly fixable problems, those who do not dramatically improve deserve further diagnostic workup.

## History-Taking

The history of the present illness is critical in determining the etiology of the mental status change. Medical history, physical examination, past history, and treatment response can lead to the diagnosis and treatment in 60% of cases of AMS. Obtaining a detailed history is often difficult if the patient is confused, cannot comply, or is unresponsive. In that situation, the provider must speak with any present family or friends about details of the mental status change, including if this was an acute or a gradual change and whether it is constant or is waxing or waning. Recent medication changes, environmental exposures, and recent travel are important areas to probe.

## Physical Examination

### Neurological

A complete neurological examination must be conducted (Figure 11.3) (3), including the Glasgow Coma Scale, signs of head trauma, mental status exam, cranial nerves, reflexes, strength, and motor function. When talking with the patient, the provider should pay attention to pressured or tangential speech, quiet speech, or inability to answer. The provider should determine if the patient is responding to internal stimuli or having visual and auditory hallucinations.

## Neurologic Examination  ☑ Check normal, circle & describe abnormal

CC & significant history: _____

Patient: _____ date: _____
Insurance: _____ (dd/mm/yr)
Date of birth: _____ M/F

**Key considerations:**  ☐ headache,  ☐ head injury,  ☐ dizziness/vertigo,  ☐ seizures,  ☐ tremors,  ☐ weakness,  ☐ incoordination,  ☐ numbness/tingling,
☐ difficulty swallowing,  ☐ difficulty speaking,  ☐ significant past history,  ☐ environmental hazards,  ☐ other: _____
☐ Refer for secondary consultation: _____
☐ Refer for diagnostic imaging: _____

### Mental Status:  ☐ WNL
**Development** (☐ good, ☐ fair, ☐ poor)
  **Behavior** (Alert, lethargic, confusion, speech)
  **Orientation** (Time, person, place & situation)
  **Memory/Concentration**
  ☐ Name president/recent newsworthy events
  ☐ 3 word or place recall at 0 and 5 minutes
  ☐ (100) - (7) up to five times (93, 86, 79...)
  ☐ Spell word backwards
☐ Draw a clock (make the time 12:30)
☐ Draw overlaping pentagons
_____
_____

### Reflexes:  ☐ WNL

| DTR (0-5) | R | L |
|---|---|---|
| Biceps (C5) | | |
| Brachioradialis (C6) | | |
| Triceps (C7) | | |
| Patella (L4) | | |
| Hamstring (L5) | | |
| Achilles (S1) | | |

| Pathologic | R | L |
|---|---|---|
| Babinski | | |
| Abdominal | | |
| Hoffman's | | |

*Note presence of clonus

### Motor Function:  ☐ WNL

| Motor (0-5) | R | L |
|---|---|---|
| Deltoid (C5, C6) (axillary) | | |
| Brachioradialis (C5, C6) (radial) | | |
| Biceps (C5, C6) (musculocut.) | | |
| Triceps (C6, C7, C8, T1) (radial) | | |
| Wrist flexors (C6, C7) (med./ulnar) | | |
| Wrist extensors (C6, C7, C8) (rad.) | | |
| Interossei (C7, C8, T1) (ulnar) | | |
| Tib. anterior (L4, L5) (deep per.) | | |
| Extensor hallicus longus (L4, L5, S1) (deep peroneal) | | |
| Fibularis (peroneus) longus (L5, S1) (superficial peroneal) | | |

### Cranial Nerves:  ☐ WNL

| I - Olfactory | R | L |
|---|---|---|
| Scent #1 | | |
| Scent #2 | | |
| **II - Optic** | | |
| Visual acuity | | |
| Visual fields | | |
| Fundiscopic exam | | |
| **III, IV, VI - Oculomotor, trochlear, abducens** | | |
| 'H' pattern | | |
| Convergence | | |
| Nystagmus | | |
| Consensual light reflex | | |
| **V - Trigeminal** | | |
| Lateral jaw deviation | | |
| Masseter contraction | | |
| Face sensation | | |
| Corneal touch reflex | | |

| VII - Facial | R | L |
|---|---|---|
| Facial expressions | | |
| Facial expression #2 | | |
| Normal eye moisture | | |
| **VIII - Vestibulocochlear** | | |
| Rhomberg's test | | |
| Auditory acuity | | |
| Weber | | |
| Rinne | | |
| **IX, X - Glossopharyngeal & Vagus** | | |
| Gag reflex | | |
| Elevation of palate | | |
| **XI - Spinal accessory** | | |
| Trapezius muscle test | | |
| SCM muscle test | | |
| **XII - Hypoglossal** | | |
| Stick out tongue | | |

### Cerebellar:  ☐ WNL

| | R | L |
|---|---|---|
| Rapid finger movement | | |
| Rapid pro/supination | | |
| Finger-to-nose/finger | | |
| Heel down shin | | |
| Holme's rebound sign | | |
| Gait/heel-toe walk | | |

### Nerve Tension:  ☐ WNL

| | R | L |
|---|---|---|
| Straight Leg Raise | | |
| Maximal SLR | | |
| Bragard's | | |
| Femoral nerve traction | | |
| Median nerve traction | | |
| Radial nerve traction | | |
| Ulnar nerve traction | | |
| Tinel's | | |

### Sensory:  ☐ WNL

| | R | L |
|---|---|---|
| Light touch | | |
| Vibration | | |
| Stereognosis | | |
| Graphesthesia | | |
| 2-pointdiscrim | | |
| Positionsense | | |
| Proprioception | | |
| Romberg | | |
| Sharp/dull | | |
| Hot/cold | | |

**DDx:**
_____
_____
_____
_____

Signature:            Date:

**FIGURE 11.3**  Neurological examination. (From Vizniak, N., *Neurologic Exam Form*, Professional Health Systems, Wilmington, IL, 2017. With permission.)

TABLE 11.1

Basic Laboratory Evaluations

| Lab Test | Possible Diagnosis |
|---|---|
| Ammonia level | Liver failure |
| Beta-hydroxybutyrate | Diabetic ketoacidosis (DKA) |
| Lactic acid | Sepsis |
| Blood alcohol level | Alcohol intoxication |
| Urine drug | Illicit substances |
| Drug level | Epilepsy |
| Troponin/cardiac enzymes | Myocardial infarction (MI) |
| Thyroid-stimulating hormone and free T4 | Thyroid storm, hypothyroidism |

## Cardiovascular

Cardiac auscultation may reveal arrhythmias and heart murmurs. The physician should auscultate over the carotid arteries to listen for bruits and assess the patient's peripheral circulation by feeling pedal pulses and checking capillary refill times.

## Abdomen/Extremities

The abdomen should be assessed by palpation to determine if the uterus feels rigid or if contractions are palpable, and it should be assessed for fundal tenderness. The abdomen is inspected for ascites, ecchymosis, rash, and excoriations. The examination of the patient's skin is not restricted to only the abdomen but should include the back and limbs, with careful attention paid to track marks, petechiae, jaundice, and pallor.

## Diagnostic Testing

The basic laboratory evaluations for pregnant women with AMS are displayed in Table 11.1. If the patient has an elevated anion gap or signs of respiratory problems, obtain an arterial blood gas to assess for respiratory or metabolic acidosis or alkalosis that can alter the mental status. If the patient is hypotensive or has electrolyte abnormalities, check the serum cortisol level to assess for adrenal insufficiency.

## Imaging

Patients presenting with focal neurological deficits, after trauma to the head, or seizures should have an immediate noncontrast head computed tomography (CT) scan. Magnetic resonance imaging (MRI) with magnetic resonance angiography (MRA) and magnetic resonance venography (MRV) is used to assess for thromboses, aneurysms, and lesions. Neurologists often order an electroencephalogram in patients presenting with seizures or patients who appear postictal.

Patients with pulmonary symptoms, including dyspnea, cough, and wheezing, should have a chest X-ray (CXR) done to look for pulmonary edema, pneumonia, pneumothorax, and more. If the patient has pleuritic chest pain, tachycardia, dyspnea, and/or hypoxia, imaging is needed to rule out pulmonary embolus.

## Causes of Acute Mental Status Change

### Neurological

In the general younger population, neurological issues are not often the source of acute mental status change; however, pregnancy-related physiological changes and specific syndromes increase the risk of neurological insult.

## Stroke

Stroke is rare in young women, but its incidence increases in pregnancy due to the hypercoagulability of pregnancy. The overall incidence is 3.5–5 women out of 100,000. The risk of stroke increases fourfold in the setting of preeclampsia (PEC). Risk factors include PEC, hypertension (HTN), prior atriovenous malformation, and aneurysm. Hallmark symptoms include severe headache, acute mental status changes, seizure, and focal neurological deficits, such as slurred speech, facial droop, and difficulty with ambulation. Noncontrast CT of the head should be done. Once the diagnosis of stroke is made, treatment must be promptly initiated. In nonhemorrhagic strokes, tissue plasminogen activator (tPA) is used within a 3-hour time frame. Data regarding the use of tPA in pregnancy are rare. The rates of maternal mortality are 1%; fetal loss, 6%; and preterm delivery, 6%. The use of tPA is controversial due to the concern for placental abruption, preterm delivery, and uterine and intracerebral fetal or maternal hemorrhage.

## Cerebral Venous Thrombosis

Pregnancy and the immediate postpartum period are the peak incident times that central venous thrombosis occurs, with a rate of 11.5 women out of 100,000. This is most likely due to the procoagulation state that pregnant women experience. The mortality rate is 9%. The most common affected areas are the superior sagittal and transverse sinuses. Headaches, seizures, mental status changes, and papilledema occur due to increased intracranial pressure. When the thrombus is within the cavernous sinus, women have cranial nerve deficits, proptosis, and painful ophthalmoplegia. Diagnosis is made by imaging with MRA and MRV. Women are treated by full anticoagulation with unfractionated or low-molecular weight heparin. Treatment is discontinued when repeat imaging demonstrates the recanalization of the previously blocked blood vessel.

## Reversible Cerebral Vasoconstrictions Syndrome

Reversible cerebral vasoconstrictions syndrome (RCVS) is a change in the cerebral vascular tone, with vasospasm on angiopathy. Risk factors include the postpartum state, a history of migraine headaches, hypertensive encephalopathy, and vasoactive medications. Women not only often describe a "thunderclap" headache but can also present with acute mental status changes, seizures, and focal neurological deficits similar to a stroke presentation. When vasospasm cannot be identified, RCVS is primarily a diagnosis of exclusion. Hypoperfusion may be seen with MRI, but watershed areas distal to the affected vessels appear completely normal. Treatment employs calcium channel blockers such as nimodipine and verapamil, glucocorticoids, and opioids to treat headache symptoms.

## Posterior Reversible Encephalopathy Syndrome

Posterior reversible encephalopathy syndrome (PRES) often occurs in the setting of PEC or eclampsia. Diffuse endothelial damage, HTN, and inflammation lead to posterior brain edema. The symptoms of PRES can slowly develop over a few days or begin acutely. Women experience headaches, confusion, seizures, and/or vision changes, including cortical blindness. PRES occurs in PEC because of the underlying endothelial damage and increased overall inflammation. CT or MRI shows symmetric edema in the parietal and occipital regions of the brain. The management of PRES involves the treatment of HTN, magnesium sulfate for seizure prophylaxis, and expedited delivery (4).

## Metabolic/Endocrine

### Electrolyte Abnormalities

Both hypo- and hypernatremia can cause mental confusion and even seizures. AMS occurs when serum sodium levels fall below 120 mEq/L or if the serum sodium level quickly decreases. Hyposmolality creates an osmolar gradient that favors water influx into cells, leading to cerebral edema. Symptoms include headache, nausea, difficulty with ambulation, confusion, seizures, obtundation, and respiratory arrest. Hyponatremia must be slowly corrected to reduce the risk of central pontine myelinolysis.

Hypernatremia can also cause AMS. The decrease in water volume in the brain can cause the rupture of cerebral vasculature. Hypernatremia is most often caused by gastrointestinal losses due to vomiting or diarrhea. Most cases are chronic and ongoing for more than 48 hours. If the urine output is excessive (greater than 5 L per day), consider lithium toxicity, primary polydipsia, hypercalcemia, central diabetes insipidus, and congenital nephrogenic diabetes insipidus. Fluid is replaced by giving 5% dextrose in water intravenously at a rate of 1.35 mL/hour × the patient's weight in kilograms.

## Diabetic Ketoacidosis

DKA results in acute mental status changes and can progress to coma and death if not corrected. DKA is usually suspected with an elevated blood glucose level in a type 1 diabetic. Rarely, DKA can occur in women with type 2 diabetes or gestational diabetes. Up to one-third of pregnant patients in DKA will present with a blood glucose level lower than 200 mg/dL (11.1 mmol/L). Workup should still be initiated in patients with a history of diabetes, AMS, and vomiting. A serum bicarbonate level lower than 18 mg/dL (2.95 mmol/L) or an anion gap higher than 10–15 mEq/L should raise suspicion for DKA despite lower blood glucose level. Arterial blood gas analysis confirms the diagnosis when the base excess exceeds −4 mEq/L.

The patient will appear acutely ill with Kussmaul breathing in order to compensate for metabolic acidosis. Urinalysis will show ketonuria and glycosuria. The patient should be immediately hydrated with normal saline. Figure 11.4 provides guidance to the treatment of DKA. Principal to this treatment is giving volume in the form of normal saline (2 L in the first 2 hours) and rapid initiation of insulin. Fetal heart monitoring often reveals signs of fetal distress. It is imperative that the mother is stabilized prior to delivery, as cesarean section can precipitate worsening of the DKA (5).

## Hyperglycemic Hyperosmolar Nonketotic Coma

Water follows glucose in the urine, causing dehydration and a hyperosmolar state. Over time, the patient cannot adequately compensate with increased fluid intake. These patients look very similar to DKA patients but do not have ketosis. Hyperglycemic hyperosmolar nonketotic (HHNK) coma initially presents with confusion and lethargy and then progresses to obtundation and coma. The management of HHNK is similar to the management of DKA. The treatment of hyperosmolar hyperglycemic state includes fluid resuscitation, correction of electrolyte imbalances, and regular insulin to correct hyperglycemia at a rate of 0.1 units/kg/hour (6).

## Thyroid

Hyperthyroidism complicates 0.2% of pregnancies, with 85% of cases attributed to Graves' disease. Undertreated or undiagnosed hyperthyroidism can lead to thyroid storm, which has a 20–30% fetal and maternal mortality rate. Thyroid storm should be suspected in a woman presenting with agitation, delirium, tremors, fevers, palpitations, and/or atrial fibrillation. Other etiologies of thyrotoxicosis include toxic adenoma, multinodular goiter, exogenous thyroid hormone use, molar pregnancy, and transient gestational hyperthyroidism. For thyroid storm, 300–600 mg propylthiouracil is immediately given by mouth. Saturated potassium iodide (two to five drops or 0.5–1 g) intravenously and beta-blockers to control tachycardia and atrial fibrillation should be considered in severe cases. The obstetrician-gynecologist should emergently consult endocrinology and cardiology in cases of thyroid storm.

Like thyroid storm, severe hypothyroidism can cause acute mental status changes in the form of myxedema coma. The treatment of myxedema coma includes IV bolus of levothyroxine (4 μg/kg of lean body weight, approximately 200–250 μg) in a single or divided dose. If adrenal insufficiency is suspected, stress doses of IV glucocorticoids must be administered (7).

## Adrenal

Patients with adrenal insufficiency may present as confused, hypotensive, weak, nauseous with vomiting, anorexic, and hyperthermia. Adrenal insufficiency may have an insidious onset with nonspecific

**Fetus**

- CEFM if viable pregnancy, doptones if pre-viable
- Often presents with category II FHT
- Oxygen
- IV fluids
- Treat mother first!
- Expect improvement after stabilizing the mother

**Fluid replacement**

- IV fluid bolus with 0.9% NaCl (1 L/hour × 2 hours)
- Change fluids to 0.45% NaCl at 250 mL/hour
- Change fluids to D5 0.45% NaCl at 250 mL/hour when blood glucose <250 mg/dL
- Continue IV fluids × 24–48 hours
- Monitor strict intake and output
- Foley catheter for accurate monitoring
- Goal urine output >50 cm³/hour

**Insulin**

- Regular insulin 10 units IV
- Insulin gtt: 0.1 units/kg/hour
- Goal: decrease blood glucose by 50 mg/dL in first hour
- When blood glucose ≤200, decrease to 0.05 units/kg/hour

**Potassium**

- Add 20–30 mEq/L of K⁺ to insulin infusion if starting serum K⁺ is between 3.3 and 5.3 mEq/L
- Goal K⁺: 4–5 mEq/L

**Underlying etiology**

- Detailed H&P, focus on past medical history and current medications, medication compliance
- Arterial blood gas, oxygen saturation monitoring
- Look for infection (urine and blood cultures, CXR, amniocentesis)

**FIGURE 11.4**  Treatment of DKA. CEFM, continuous electronic fetal monitoring; FHT, fetal heart tracing; GGT, drip (ggt); H&P, History and Physical.

symptoms confused for normal pregnancy symptoms. Physical examination reveals bronze areas of skin, particularly on the elbows, blue-black discoloration on mucosal surfaces, and diminished axillary and pubic hair. Stressors such as infection, labor, dehydration, and trauma can precipitate adrenal crisis. Adrenal insufficiency should be strongly suspected if the patient has risk factors such as another auto-immune disease (hypothyroidism, pernicious anemia, type 1 diabetes) or prior corticosteroid use and electrolyte abnormalities. Women in adrenal crisis will be hyponatremic and hyperkalemic. Treatment is with 100 mg hydrocortisone intravenously every 6 hours for 24 hours. This dose is slowly tapered and converted to an oral maintenance dose after 4–5 days. This is a high enough dose that there are miner-alocorticoid effects, so a mineralocorticoid does not need to be administered. Replete fluids and glucose.

## Toxins and Drugs

The ingestion of toxins, illegal substances, and medications is a common cause of AMS in the emergency room. Substance abuse is common in pregnant patients with 10–15% of women admitting use at some time during their pregnancy.

## Opioids

Naloxone (Narcan) should be quickly administered in a patient presenting with acute mental status changes associated with miosis, depressed respiratory rate (less than 12 breaths per minute), or circumstantial evidence of opioid use. Administer 2 mg intravenously. The onset of action is within 1–3 minutes. The dose can be repeated if there is no response in 3–5 minutes. The provider should ensure that they have a backup team in the room during administration, as the patient can become violent and acutely combative during the opioid overdose reversal.

## Benzodiazepines

Flumazenil should be given to women with suspected or known benzodiazepine use. However, benzodiazepines should not be reversed if used to control life-threatening conditions such as elevated intracranial pressure or epilepsy. The initial dose is 0.2 mg intravenously over 30 seconds. If there is no response, administer 0.3 mg intravenously. The total dose of 5 mg should not be exceeded.

## Alcohol

Both alcohol intoxication and withdrawal can cause AMS. Intoxicated women present with euphoria incoordination, AMS, and even aggressive behavior. If overdose is severe, depressant effects are seen, including bradycardia, hypotension, and respiratory depression. Lab work includes liver function and blood alcohol level tests. Administer 100 mg thiamine intravenously followed by dextrose-containing fluids. The onset of withdrawal occurs within 6–60 hours. Withdrawal symptoms can be seen even more quickly in pregnant women as alcohol metabolism is increased during pregnancy. Short-acting benzodiazepines are given on a tapered schedule. The rate of maternal or fetal mortality is 10–15% if untreated and 1–2% if treated (8).

## Sympathomimetics

Sympathomimetics include cocaine, amphetamines, and ephedrines (constituents of cold medications). They cause HTN due to vasoconstriction. Due to its stimulant activity, women present with AMS best characterized by agitation and even frank psychosis. Patients are tachycardic, hypertensive, hyperthermic, and tachypneic. Severe complications include placental abruption, hypertensive urgency followed by multiorgan dysfunction, pulmonary edema, and even death due to circulatory collapse. Cocaine use can be diagnosed with a urine drug screen. Supportive measures must be initiated, and both mother and fetus should be monitored for at least 24 hours. No antidote exists. During pregnancy, the safest sedating medications include antihistamines and benzodiazepines, but only at the lowest dose needed.

## Anticholinergics

Women can present with anticholinergic toxicity by overingesting anticholinergics, antihistamines, antipsychotics with anticholinergic properties, and cyclic antidepressants with anticholinergic properties. Drug reactions can occur when, for example, an anticholinergic is taken along with an antihistamine. Symptoms include flushing, edema, AMS, hyperthermia, dry skin and mucus membranes, tachycardia, urinary retention, and tremors. Medication reconciliation and patient history-taking is key in diagnosis. If the patient is febrile, blood and urine cultures should be obtained. Blood work includes complete metabolic panel, creatinine kinase to rule out rhabdomyolysis, and arterial blood gas. A 12-lead electrocardiogram should be obtained as conduction abnormalities can occur. Treatment includes activated charcoal if ingestion was recent. Treatment is otherwise supportive.

## Carbon Monoxide

Carbon monoxide poisoning occurs in improperly ventilated areas. Symptoms include headache, dyspnea, dizziness, chest pain, confusion, impaired judgment, Cheyne–Stokes respirations, and visual disturbances. Due to lack of oxygenation, renal failure, pulmonary edema, blindness, and MI can occur. Carbon monoxide crosses the placenta and has even higher affinity for fetal hemoglobin. Carbon monoxide poisoning must thus be aggressively treated in pregnancy. One hundred percent oxygen is administered via a nonrebreathing mask. If carbon monoxide saturation is greater than 15% or if AMS is present, hyperbaric oxygen is needed.

## Infectious Diseases

Infection may cause AMS, either specifically from encephalitis or meningitis or more generally as a manifestation of sepsis. The current understanding of sepsis is that of organ dysfunction associated with infection. One of the cardinal clinical markers of this organ dysfunction is an AMS.

### Meningitis and Encephalitis

Meningitis is an inflammatory disease of the leptomeninges that surround the brain and spinal cord. The most common organisms in adults are *Streptococcus pneumoniae* and *Neisseria meningitidis*. The classic triad of symptoms is mental status change, fever, and nuchal rigidity. Most patients have elevated temperatures, typically higher than 38.0°C. Many patients complain of a diffuse headache. Patients with suspected meningitis should have immediate blood cultures drawn and lumbar puncture, following CT imaging of the head to ensure that there is no large mass lesion causing increased intracranial pressure.

## Trauma

Trauma occurs in 6–7% of pregnancies, with more than half of obstetric trauma caused by motor vehicle collisions. Head trauma often manifests as AMS. More than 50% of trauma-related mortality is due to head trauma. As with any trauma, the primary survey is conducted first. Stable patients must have a CT scan of the head to quickly look for lesions, bleeding, and infarction.

## Renal

Renal failure results in the accumulation of urea and other toxins. This uremia clinically manifests as slowed cognition, drowsiness, and mild agitation. As renal failure progresses, patients are disoriented and confused and act bizarrely. Patients later develop seizure and stupor and can enter coma. Lab work shows markedly elevated creatinine and blood urea nitrogen. Complete metabolic panels and electrolytes should be obtained, as many patients with kidney failure have electrolyte derangement. Calcium, phosphate, and parathyroid hormone levels should be obtained as patients with kidney disease can develop secondary hyperparathyroidism. These patients have worsening mental status due to a combination of uremia and elevated calcium levels. Uremic encephalopathy is an indication for dialysis. The AMS is reversible with treatment.

## Pregnancy-Specific

### Eclampsia

New-onset seizure and the postictal state that follows are common causes of AMS during pregnancy (9). When seizures occur in the setting of elevated blood pressures (≥140 mmHg systolic and/or ≥90 mmHg diastolic) beyond 20 weeks, eclampsia must be considered. Laboratory derangements (elevated creatinine and liver function tests, low platelet count, and/or signs of hemolysis with elevated lactate dehydrogenase, uric acid, and schistocytes on peripheral blood smear) and proteinuria should also be assessed. Eclamptic seizures occur in 1–2% of women with PEC. Patients often have headaches and vision changes, including blurred vision and photophobia, prior to seizure onset. Physical examination will reveal hyperreflexia and clonus. Eclamptic seizures occur when uncontrolled HTN causes cerebral autoregulation failure, with an increased intracranial pressure and extracellular edema. Others speculate that the brain overregulates, which causes brain hypoperfusion and subsequent seizure activity.

Acute treatment is the administration of 4–6 g of magnesium sulfate pushed intravenously for over 20 minutes, followed by 2 g/hour unless the patient has pulmonary edema, renal failure, or signs of magnesium toxicity. If IV access has not been established, intramuscular injections of 10 g magnesium sulfate should be administered (5 g intramuscularly in each buttock). Patients who have had unwitnessed seizures will often be confused with AMS.

## Acute Fatty Liver Disease of Pregnancy

Acute fatty liver disease is a rare disease, complicating 1 out of 10,000–15,000 pregnancies. The maternal mortality rate is 18%. Mortality is caused by lipid accumulation in the liver, pancreas, kidneys, brain, and bone marrow. Liver failure occurs due to hyperammonemia and fatty necrosis. Women die due to fulminant hepatic failure, encephalopathy, renal failure, pulmonary edema, and coagulopathy. The disease gradually develops with nonspecific complaints, including nausea, vomiting, abdominal pain, and tachycardia. The disease progresses until the patient has jaundice, right upper quadrant pain, vomiting, and headache. Severe disease manifests with acute mental status change due to elevated ammonia levels. Laboratory testing reveals elevated bilirubin, liver function tests, abnormal coagulation factors, and hypoglycemia. Liver transaminases are mildly increased, usually between 100 and 1000 units/L. Bilirubin is typically higher than 5 mg/dL. Ammonia levels are elevated. Fifty percent of women with acute fatty liver of pregnancy have symptoms of PEC, including HTN, proteinuria, neurological symptoms, and right upper quadrant pain. However, neurological symptoms rapidly manifest and can progress to confusion, agitation, asterixis, psychosis, and seizures. Treatment includes the stabilization of HTN, hypoglycemia, and coagulopathy followed by rapid delivery. Neomycin is administered at a dose of 6–12 g per day to reduce further formation of ammonia by gut microflora. Typically, the disease worsens in the first 2 days postpartum and then gradually improves. Permanent renal dysfunction can occur. If the mental status deteriorates or there is persistent coagulopathy, plasmapheresis can be done (Table 11.2) (10–13).

## Hematologic

### Acute Intermittent Porphyria

Acute intermittent porphyria (AIP) is a genetic disease with an autosomal dominant inheritance pattern. Women with AIP are deficient in porphobilinogen deaminase (PBG), an enzyme in the heme breakdown pathway. There is often low expressivity of the disorder until there is an exacerbating stressor, such as labor. The biggest risk factor for a flare of AIP is the use of medications that induce hepatic cytochrome p450 activity. While AIP is often quiet during pregnancy, the use of medications such as metoclopramide (commonly used to treat pregnancy-related nausea and headaches) and conditions that stress the body, such as hyperemesis gravidarum, can induce an attack. Neurological dysfunction manifests as extreme anxiety, acute mental status changes, and mental deterioration due to the neurotoxic effects of accumulated porphyrin. Abdominal pain occurs in 85–90% of attacks. Patients are usually tachycardic, hypertensive, restless, and diaphoretic.

Porphyrins build up in the system and are renally excreted. Women undergoing flares have reddish-brown urine. The urine levels of PBG and delta-aminolevulinic acid are elevated. For mild attacks, glucose loading is the treatment of choice in order to downregulate the hepatic enzyme delta-aminolevulinic acid synthase 1, which is involved in heme biosynthesis. In severe attacks, characterized by severe mental status changes or psychosis, IV hemin is used (14).

### Thrombotic Thrombocytopenic Purpura

Thrombotic thrombocytopenic purpura (TTP) is a rare disease that presents as a triad of thrombocytopenia, microangiopathic hemolytic anemia, and neurological changes. These signs are present in 75% of patients with TTP. In 33% of patients, patients additionally have fever and acute renal failure. Diagnostic testing shows severe thrombocytopenia with platelets less than 50,000, anemia with hemoglobin less

**TABLE 11.2**

Differential Diagnosis and Complications of Acute Fatty Liver of Pregnancy

| Disease State | Initial Signs and Symptoms | Later Signs and Symptoms | Laboratory Abnormalities | Maternal Complications and Comments |
|---|---|---|---|---|
| Acute fatty liver of pregnancy | Malaise, epigastric pain, nausea/ vomiting, jaundice | Encephalopathy, renal failure, DIC, hypoglycemia | Elevated white blood cell count; elevated ALT, AST, and bilirubin; normal LDH; low platelet count | Pancreatitis, diabetes insipidus, fulminant hepatic failure, sepsis; may also have HELLP syndrome |
| Severe PEC | Headache, right upper quadrant pain, edema, HTN | Hypertensive emergency, pulmonary edema | Mildly elevated ALT, proteinuria | Eclampsia, acute renal failure, hepatic capsular rupture |
| HELLP syndrome | Right upper quadrant pain, nausea/vomiting, malaise, headaches, visual changes | Hematuria, petechiae, ecchymosis | Low platelet count, elevated bilirubin, elevated AST, ALT, LDH | DIC, acute renal failure, hepatic hemorrhage or failure, ARDS, sepsis, cerebrovascular accident |
| Viral hepatitis | Nausea, vomiting, fever, jaundice | Encephalopathy, sepsis, coagulopathy, hypoglycemia | Very elevated transaminases, elevated bilirubin, positive serology | Fulminant hepatic failure, hepatic coma, sepsis, GI bleeding |
| TTP | Mild fever, nausea/ vomiting, abdominal pain, petechiae | CNS effects— headache, visual changes, confusion, seizures; other organ involvement | Very low platelet count and hematocrit, very elevated LDH and bilirubin, mildly elevated ALT, AST | Diffuse subcortical microvascular disease, acute renal failure; could cause placental thrombosis |
| Antiphospholipid antibody syndrome | Thrombosis | Thrombotic renal disease, GI ischemia | Low hematocrit and platelet count, presence of LA, aCL, or $\beta_2$-GP-I | Multiorgan failure leading to "catastrophic antiphospholipid syndrome," development of TTP |

*Source:* Kelsey, J. J., *Obstetric Emergencies in the ICU: PSAP-VII: Critical and Urgent Care*, American College of Clinical Pharmacy, Lenexa, KS, 2010. With permission; from Ko, H. H., and Yoshida, E., *Canadian Journal of Gastroenterology*, 20, 25–30, 2006; Sibai, B. M., *Obstetrics and Gynecology*, 109, 4, 956–966, 2007.

*Note:* acL, anticardiolipin antibodies; ALT, alanine aminotransferase; ARDS, adult respiratory distress syndrome; AST, aspartate aminotransferase; $\beta_2$-GP-I, $\beta_2$-glycoprotein-I antibodies; CNS, central nervous system; DIC, disseminated intravascular coagulation; GI, gastrointestinal; HELLP, hemolysis, elevated liver enzymes, and low platelet count; LA, lupus anticoagulant; LDH, lactate dehydrogenase; TTP, thrombotic thrombocytopenic purpura.

than 10, elevated creatinine, elevated unconjugated bilirubin, hematuria and proteinuria, and decreased ADAMTS13 level. Patients are treated with plasmapheresis until remission (15).

*Antiphospholipid Antibody Syndrome*

Women with antiphospholipid syndrome (APLS) can develop thromboses, which may lead to transient ischemic attacks and ischemic strokes. In addition, patients with APLS can have white matter brain lesions that cause mild to severe cognitive deficits and functional impairments. These vasculopathic patients can be managed with aspirin. Rarely, the syndrome presents with multiorgan failure due to vascular thromboses. This catastrophic type of APLS occurs in 0.8% of women with the syndrome, but with a fatality rate of up to 50%. In women presenting with catastrophic APLS, treatment must begin before

TABLE 11.3

Differential Indicators for Organic versus Functional Cause of Problems

| | Organic | Functional/Psychiatric |
|---|---|---|
| History | Acute onset | Slower onset (weeks to months) |
| Mental status exam | • Waxing and waning consciousness | • Alert |
| | • Disoriented | • Oriented |
| | • Memory impairment | • Memory impairment |
| | • Hallucinations | • Hallucinations (typically auditory) |
| | • Cognitive impairment | • Delusions |
| | • Lack of attention | • Agitation |
| Physical exam | • Abnormal vital signs | • Normal vital signs |
| | • Focal neurological deficits | • No neurological deficits |
| | • Signs of trauma | • No signs of trauma |

awaiting test results if suspicion is high based on prior history. Antibody testing includes anticardiolipin immunoglobulin G (IgG) and immunoglobulin M (IgM), anti-beta-2-glycoprotein IgG and IgM, lupus anticoagulant with dilute Russell viper venom time, and activated partial thromboplastin time. The management of catastrophic APLS includes anticoagulation due to thrombotic disease, glucocorticoids to suppress the immune system and reduce cytokine formation, plasma exchange, and IV immunoglobulin to remove anticardiolipin antibodies.

## Psychiatric

Patients with psychiatric illnesses can present with mental status changes. It is critical to determine if the AMS is due to an organic or psychiatric problem. The obstetrician-gynecologist should not assume that mental status change is due to a psychiatric issue even in a patient with psychiatric illness. Workup should always be aimed at ruling out the most dangerous causes first.

Patient interview can provide many clues and details. Attention should be paid to the patient's overall appearance (unkempt, bizarre clothing, posture) and style of speech (pressured speech, disorganized thinking). The provider should attempt to determine if the patient is responding to internal stimuli. If a psychiatric problem is suspected, one must assess for suicidal and homicidal ideation. See further Table 11.3.

## Summary

There is a wide differential for AMS. Obstetricians are the frontline providers for pregnant women and must have the knowledge of causes and management strategies for AMS. This chapter provides a framework to guide both rapid treatment and deductive reasoning. Familiarity with the common presentations and causes of AMS allows the physician to care for both mother and fetus competently and safely.

## REFERENCES

1. Belfort MA, Saade GR, Foley MR, Phelan JP, Dildy GA. *Critical care obstetrics*, 5th ed. Hoboken, NJ: Wiley-Blackwell; 2010.
2. Resnik R, Creasy RK, Iams JD, Lockwood CJ, Moore T, Greene MF. *Creasy and Resnik's maternal-fetal medicine: Principles and practice.* 7th ed. Philadelphia, PA: Saunders; 2014.
3. Vizniak N. *Neurologic exam form.* Wilmington, IL: Professional Health Systems; 2017.
4. Hosley CM, McCullough LD. Acute neurological issues in pregnancy and peripartum. *Neurohospitalist* 2011; 1(2):104-116.
5. De Veciana M. Diabetes ketoacidosis in pregnancy. *Semin Perinatol* 2013; 37(4):267-273.

6. Gonzalez JM, Edlow AG, Silber A, Elovitz MA. Hyperosmolar hyperglycemic state of pregnancy with intrauterine fetal demise and preeclampsia. *Am J Perinatol* 2007; 24(9):541-543.

7. Singh N, Tripathi R, Mala YM, Verma D. Undiagnosed hypothyroidism in pregnancy leading to myxedema coma in labor: Diagnosing and managing this rare emergency. *J Preg Child Health* 2016; 3(2):1-2.

8. Myrick H, Anton RF. Treatment of alcohol withdrawal. *Alcohol Health Res World* 1998; 22(1):38-43.

9. Gabbe SG, Niebyl JR, Simpson JL. *Obstetrics: Normal and problem pregnancies.* 3rd ed. New York: Churchill Livingstone; 1996.

10. Kelsey JJ. *Obstetric emergencies in the ICU: PSAP-VII: Critical and urgent care.* Lenexa, KS: American College of Clinical Pharmacy; 2010.

11. Ko HH, Yoshida E. Acute fatty liver of pregnancy. *Can J Gastroenterol* 2006; 20:25-30.

12. Sibai BM, Imitators of severe preeclampsia. *Obstet Gynecol*, 2007; 109:956-966.

13. Pandey CK, Karna ST, Pandey VK, Tandon M. Acute liver failure in pregnancy: Challenges and management. *Indian J Anaesth* 2015; 59(3):144-149.

14. Marsden JT, Rees DC. A retrospective analysis of outcome of pregnancy in patients with acute porphyria. *J Inherit Metab Dis* 2010; 33(5):591-596.

15. Scully M, Thomas M, Underwood M, Watson H, Langley K, Camilleri RS et al. Thrombotic thrombocytopenic purpura and pregnancy: Presentation, management, and subsequent pregnancy outcomes. *Blood* 2014;124(2):211-219.

# 12

## Fever

**Anna Maya Powell, MD**

### CONTENTS

## Definition

Fever is neither necessary nor specific as a marker of infection, but it commonly accompanies infection.

*Fever in pregnancy* has been suspected to contribute to adverse pregnancy outcomes. The strongest evidence in the literature (1) suggests that fever in the first trimester increases risk for neural tube defects, congenital heart defects, and oral cleft 1.5–3-fold (1).

Fever or hyperthermia at any point in pregnancy, however, should be considered a symptom, not a diagnosis. As such, it is important to generate an appropriate differential diagnosis to guide lab test and imaging modalities to help reach a correct diagnosis. Fever is generally defined as a temperature that is ≥100.4°F or 38.0°C. The timing of fever and associated signs and symptoms in pregnancy should also be used to guide the differential diagnosis. Infectious and noninfectious causes of fever should be considered; however, the clinical spectrum of sepsis should be identified as soon as possible to decrease maternal and fetal morbidity and mortality.

## Clinical Spectrum of Sepsis in Obstetrics

It is important to be familiar with the clinical spectrum of sepsis and its range of manifestations. Definitions of sepsis and septic shock were recently revised by the Third International Consensus for Sepsis and Septic Shock task force. The specific physiological parameters do not take into account normal physiological changes of pregnancy, so alternative criteria have been proposed, including the Sepsis in Obstetrics Score (SOS) (2), the Modified Early Warning Score or the Rapid Emergency Medicine

Understand normal maternal physiologic
changes in pregnancy

• Normal temperature range: 36–38.4
• Respiratory rate (RR): 12–24
• Heart rate (HR): ≤119
• PaCO2: <32 mmHg
• WBC count: 5.7–16.9/uL

(a)

Identify sepsis

• Sepsis-3 guidelines: for ICU encounter, consider using the
sepsis organ failure assessment score (SOFA)[1] = PaO2/FiO2
ratio, Glasgow coma scale (GCS) score, mean arterial
pressure (mmHg), administration of vasopressors with
type/dose/infusion rate, serum creatinine (mg/dL) or urine
output (mL/d), bilirubin (mg/dL) and platelet count ($10^9$/uL)
• A SOFA score >2 was associated with an in-hospital
mortality >10%
• For non ICU encounter, consider use of "quick" SOFA or
qSOFA score[2] = respiratory rate (breath/min), GCS scare,
systolic BP (mmHg)
• **Consider use of SOS score  as SOFA and qSOFA not
validated for pregnancy

(b)

Start broad empiric treatment
Narrow to target most likely source for infection
Consider non-infectious sources

• Cover for suspected source: bacterial-clindamycin with
aminoglycoside (guntupalli)
• Vancomycin (MRSA) and piperacillin-tazobactam (gram
positive and gram negative coverage)
• Consider antifungal or antiviral coverage depending on
suspected infection source

(c)

[1] Seymour et al. demonstrated predictive validity of SOFA score with AUROC = 0.74; 95% CI 0.73-0.76 in a
large retrospective cohort (3).
[2] Seymour et al. demonstrated predictive validity of qSOFA score with AUROC = 0.81; 95% CI 0.8-0.82 in a
large retrospective cohort (3).

FIGURE 12.1   Key points—approach to sepsis. (a) Understand normal maternal physiologic changes in pregnancy.
(b) Identify sepsis. (c) Approach to treatment of sepsis. (From Bauer, M. E. et al., Maternal physiologic parameters in relationship to systemic inflammatory response syndrome criteria, *Obstetrics and Gynecology*, 124, 3, 535–41, 2014; Singer, M. et al.,
*Journal of the American Medical Association*, 315, 801–10, 2016; Seymour, C. W. et al., *Journal of the American Medical
Association*, 315, 762–74, 2016; Shankar-Hari, M. et al., *Journal of the American Medical Association*, 315, 775–87, 2016.)

Score; Albright et al. (2) showed a sensitivity of 88.9% and specificity of 99.2% and a positive predictive value of 16.7% compared to 4.6% and 11.1%, respectively, when applying a retrospective cohort
of pregnant and postpartum women using SOS compared to the other two scoring systems. A cutoff of
≥6 was used, and these women were more likely to be admitted to the intensive care unit (ICU) or telemetry
unit and have positive blood cultures, fetal tachycardia, and longer duration of hospitalization than those
with an SOS score of <6. An example of a general approach to the obstetric patient with suspected sepsis
is outlined in Figure 12.1 (3–6).

## Incidence and Mortality

About 200–700 women per 100,000 deliveries require ICU admission (7). Sepsis accounts for 5–8% of
ICU admissions in pregnancy (8). Pregnant women may undergo rapid progression from initial sepsis

recognition to the development of severe sepsis (9). In the United States, infection or sepsis accounted for 12.7% of pregnancy-related deaths in 2011–2012. The Centers for Disease Control monitor pregnancy-related deaths and reported a higher pregnancy-related mortality ratio during 2009–2011 related to infection and sepsis deaths. In 2009–2010, influenza A (H1N1) pmd09 pandemic occurred in the United States, and influenza deaths accounted for 12% of all pregnancy-related deaths during that time (10). A systematic analysis by the World Health Organization reported that sepsis caused 10.7% of maternal deaths between 2003 and 2009 and that hemorrhage, hypertensive disorders, and sepsis caused over half of maternal deaths worldwide collectively (11).

## Generating the Differential Diagnosis

### Identify Potential System Source and Assess for Additional Risk Factors

As many serious global health concerns continue to transcend physical and territorial boundaries, it becomes imperative to take *a proper travel history* from patients as part of a thorough history and physical examination. In 2015, the Zika and Ebola viruses both caught worldwide attention; although the Zika virus is under further investigation regarding its association with microcephaly, and the most recent Ebola outbreak demonstrated high morbidity and mortality in pregnant and nonpregnant persons alike. Travel history should include the destination and if the patient was given appropriate prophylaxis. A review of travel and routine health vaccinations may be pertinent. Additionally, it is important to distinguish the timing of symptoms before or after travel.

Emergent noninfectious causes associated with fever should also be considered in the acutely ill patient. A brief history and physical exam will help place the symptoms into context.

Neuroleptic malignant syndrome is a potentially fatal tetrad of "mental status changes, extrapyramidal symptoms, hyperpyrexia and autonomic instability" developing after the use of antipsychotics, as well as nonneuroleptic agents with antidopinergic activity such as metoclopramide or promethazine (12,13). While it may occur in 0.02–3.2% of patients using conventional antipsychotics, it is rarely reported in pregnancy (13). Treatment typically involves the discontinuation of the offending agent and supportive care to maintain cardiorespiratory parameters. Psychiatric consultation is recommended, as it may not be feasible to completely discontinue all antipsychotics for a pregnant patient with acute psychosis. Other diagnoses to consider with similar presentations include acute drug intoxication or withdrawal syndromes, serotonin syndrome, and lethal catatonia (13).

Thyroid storm is a rare complication of hyperthyroidism in 1–5% of cases (14). This medical emergency carries a mortality rate of 8–25%. Typical disease triggers include medication noncompliance or discontinuation and infection; trauma, stress, and pregnancy may also precipitate this event. Hyperthyroidism is diagnosed in 5.9 per 1000 pregnant women per year in the United States. Treatment involves supportive measures, antithyroid drugs, iodine administration, beta-blockers, glucocorticoids, and the identification of the underlying illness that triggered the thyroid storm (14).

Diabetic ketoacidosis (DKA) is a medical emergency occurring in the setting of diabetes mellitus. Pregnancy is a risk factor for DKA and can make the diagnosis more challenging. Medication noncompliance and preceding viral or bacterial infections are thought to be triggers. DKA is characterized by hyperglycemia and ketosis and dehydration. DKA can lead to adverse perinatal outcomes including fetal demise, likely due to hypoxic insult. The mainstay of treatment revolves around volume replacement and the correction of maternal acidosis (15).

## Antenatal Conditions Causing Fever

The antenatal conditions causing fever are illustrated in Figure 12.2, with their timing shown in Table 12.1. The approach to management is shown in Figure 12.3, with differential diagnosis by prevalence in Table 12.2.

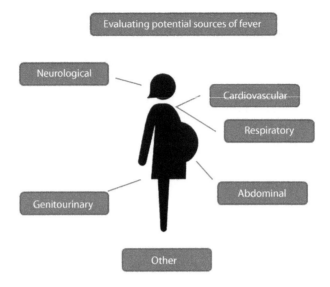

FIGURE 12.2    Antenatal conditions causing fever.

TABLE 12.1

Timing of Fever in Pregnancy

| Antenatal Sources of Fever | Intrapartum Sources of Fever | Postpartum Sources of Fever |
| --- | --- | --- |
| **Neurological**: Meningitis, NMS, serotonin syndrome, drug intoxication, drug withdrawal, psychosis | | Atelectasis |
| **CV**: Sepsis, infective endocarditis | | Mastitis |
| **Pulmonary**: Pneumonia, tuberculosis | | Endomyometritis |
| **GI**: Gastroenteritis, infectious diarrhea, appendicitis, cholecystitis, pancreatitis, listeriosis, Clostridium difficile | Epidural anesthesia | Surgical site infection |
| **GU**: Cystitis, pyelonephritis, herpes simplex virus, acute HIV, toxic shock syndrome/Group A streptococcal infecton | Prostaglandins for labor induction | Urinary tract infection |
| **Infectious**: Influenza, TORCH, Varicella-Zoster, malaria, hemorrhagic fevers, Zika | Chorioamnionitis | Drug fever |
| **Endocrine**: Hyperthyroidism/thyroid storm, diabetic ketoacidosis | Retained products of conception/septic abortion | Venous thromboembolism |
| **Connective tissue**: Systemic Lupus Erythematosus flare | | Septic pelvic thrombophlebitis |

*Note:*  CV, cardiovascular; GI, gastrointestinal; GU, genitourinary; NMS, neuroleptic malignant syndrome; PULM, pulmonary.

## Neurological

1. Meningitis: Bacterial (*Streptococcus pneumoniae, Listeria monocytogenes*) or viral (enteroviruses, mumps, measles, influenza, arboviruses such as West Nile virus, herpes viruses)

   a.  Associated symptoms: Fever, headache, neck stiffness, nausea, emesis, altered mental status, photophobia

   b.  Risk factors: Not previously vaccinated, recent otitis or sinusitis, primary herpes simplex virus (HSV) or varicella zoster virus (VZV) diagnosis, sick contact to influenza or varicella

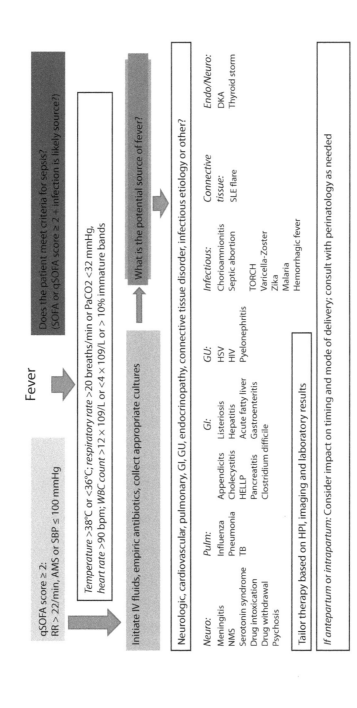

**Fever**

Does the patient meet criteria for sepsis? (SOFA or qSOFA score ≥ 2 + infection is likely source?)

qSOFA score ≥ 2:
RR > 22/min, AMS or SBP ≤ 100 mmHg

*Temperature* >38°C or <36°C; *respiratory rate* >20 breaths/min or PaCO2 <32 mmHg; *heart rate* >90 bpm; *WBC count* >12 × 109/L or <4 × 109/L or >10% immature bands

Initiate IV fluids, empiric antibiotics, collect appropriate cultures

What is the potential source of fever?

Neurologic, cardiovascular, pulmonary, GI, GU, endocrinopathy, connective tissue disorder, infectious etiology or other?

*Neuro:*
Meningitis
NMS
Serotonin syndrome
Drug intoxication
Drug withdrawal
Psychosis

*Pulm:*
Influenza
Pneumonia
TB

*GI:*
Appendicits
Cholecystitis
HELLP
Pancreatitis
Clostridium difficile

Listeriosis
Hepatitis
Acute fatty liver
Gastroenteritis

*GU:*
HSV
HIV
Pyelonephritis

*Infectious:*
Chorioamnionitis
Septic abortion

TORCH
Varicella-Zoster
Zika
Malaria
Hemorrhagic fever

*Connective tissue:*
SLE flare

*Endo/Neuro:*
DKA
Thyroid storm

Tailor therapy based on HPI, imaging and laboratory results

*If antepartum or intrapartum:* Consider impact on timing and mode of delivery; consult with perinatology as needed

FIGURE 12.3  Approach to fever in pregnancy. AMS, altered mental status; bpm, beats per minute; GI, gastrointestinal; GU, genitourinary; qSOFA, quick SOFA; SBP, systolic blood pressure.

TABLE 12.2

Differential Diagnosis of Fever (Infectious) by Prevalence

| Least Common | Less Common | Most Common |
|---|---|---|
| CV: infective carditis | | Chorioamnitis |
| Neurological: meningitis | Gastrointestinal: cheocystitis | Gastrointestinal: appendicitis |
| | Genitourinary: acute HIV, HSV | Genitourinary: pyelonephritis |
| | Pulmonary: tuberculosis | Pulmonary: pneumonia |

c. Diagnostic workup: Head CT scan to evaluate for increased intracranial pressure prior to lumbar puncture, followed by lumbar puncture. Blood cultures may also be warranted.

d. Summary: Bacterial meningitis has an annual incidence of four to six cases per 100,000 adults and results in approximately 135,000 deaths worldwide (16). The incidence of meningitis caused by *Haemophilus influenza B* has decreased with vaccination, and currently the most common causative organism is *S. pneumoniae* with a fatality rate reported as 19–37% (5,16). The most common causative organisms are *S. pneumoniae* and *L. monocytogenes* and carry a *high associated mortality rate* (17,18).

e. Treatment: Antibiotic therapy should not be delayed if lumbar puncture cannot be performed early, but once started, the sterilization of cerebrospinal fluid cultures may occur within 2 hours for *Neisseria meningitidis* and 4 hours for *S. pneumoniae* infections. Empiric antibiotic coverage should include a third-generation cephalosporin (generally, category B) and vancomycin (category C). If *Listeria* is suspected, antibiotic coverage should include ampicillin (category B). If a viral etiology is suspected, such as herpes simplex or varicella, acyclovir should be administered (category B).

## Cardiovascular

1. Sepsis
   a. See previous section on obstetric sepsis
   b. Infective endocarditis (IE)
2. Associated symptoms: Fever, chills, anorexia, weight loss, dyspnea
3. Risk factors: Intravenous (IV) drug use, nonnative heart valve, poor dentition, recent dental or surgical procedure
4. Diagnostic workup: Electrocardiogram, transthoracic echocardiogram, blood cultures
5. Summary: IE is an extremely rare event in pregnancy (0.0006% of pregnancy), but maternal mortality can reach 35% with deaths typically related to heart failure or embolic event. The associated fetal mortality rate can reach 29% (19,20).

## Respiratory

Differential diagnosis and associated symptoms

1. Pneumonia (*viral*: influenza, respiratory syncytial virus; *bacterial*: *S. pneumoniae*)
   a. Associated symptoms: Bacterial: *high fever, cough, purulent sputum production*, dyspnea, headache, fatigue, myalgias, sweat, and nausea. Atypical bacterial: dry cough, extrapulmonary manifestations (myocarditis, pericarditis, vasculitis, thrombosis) (21).

b. Risk factors: Asthma, cigarette smoking, malnutrition, liver disease, chronic obstructive pulmonary disease and pregnancy (22), alcohol or drug use, recent sick contacts, immunocompromised states (human immunodeficiency virus [HIV]).

c. Diagnostic workup: Chest X-ray (CXR) findings suggestive of pneumonia may include lobar consolidation, cavitation, and pleural effusion; viral pneumonias may present with nodular or alveolar patterns and may be more diffuse. Additionally, complete blood count, electrolytes, assessment of oxygenation status, sputum, and blood cultures should be collected, particularly if there is a clinical concern for sepsis. Rapid serological testing for influenza A and B may be reasonable. Respiratory viral panels (polymerase chain reaction [PCR] testing) may also be helpful in narrowing the differential diagnosis.

d. Summary: Pneumonia complicates 0.5–1.5 per 1000 pregnancies in the United States (22). The most common causative organism is *S. pneumoniae*, identified in 15–20% of community-acquired pneumonia cases in pregnancy. Fungal and viral organisms are also responsible for pneumonias in pregnancy, and a causative organism is identified in 40–60% of cases. Mortality rates for pregnant women with pneumonia have drastically decreased with the use of appropriate antimicrobial therapy and intensive care services (22). Bacterial pneumonia accounts for 60–80% of community-acquired pneumonia, 10–20% with atypical bacteria and 10–15% is viral; fungal pneumonias are rare in immunocompetent hosts.

e. Treatment: Initial antimicrobial choice is often empiric and should factor in considerations for common local causes of community-acquired pneumonia, local antibiotic resistance profiles, the patients comorbid conditions, and recent antibiotic usage. The Infectious Disease Society of America recommends starting with macrolide monotherapy in otherwise healthy pregnant women without recent antibiotic exposure; women meeting sepsis criteria should be started on a B-lactam (preferably amoxicillin or amoxicillin–clavulanate with alternatives of third-generation cephalosporins) in addition to a macrolide. The coverage for other organisms such as methicillin-resistant *Staphylococcus aureus* or *Pseduomonas* should be adjusted as needed.

2. Tuberculosis (*Mycobacterium tuberculosis*)

a. Associated symptoms: Productive cough, night sweats, hemoptysis

b. Risk factors: Incarceration, residence in endemic area, sick contacts, immunocompromised state (HIV)

c. Diagnostic workup: Purified protein derivative placement is a useful diagnostic tool for latent tuberculosis (TB); in the setting of active pulmonary TB, it may be falsely negative. Interferon gamma release assays (IGRAs) are comparable to tuberculin skin tests (TSTs) and may be used during pregnancy; in low incidence settings, an IGRA may be more specific and less sensitive than TST (23). CXR with abdominal shielding should be performed for positive TB skin test or IGRA result.

d. Summary: The estimated prevalence for latent TB infection (LTBI) is 14–48% based on tuberculin skin testing in the United States. In one study, Asian-American women had an odds ratio (OR) of 3.15 (95% CI: 1.62–6.14) of TB skin test positivity related to white women and an OR of 1.55 (95% CI: 1.35–1.8) compared to Hispanic women (23). HIV-infected women have a higher prevalence of LTBI and should be offered treatment in pregnancy. Differentiating between active and latent TB infection is critical. The treatment of HIV-negative women with LTBI may be deferred until postpartum, but HIV-positive women with LTBI should be offered therapy during pregnancy.

e. Treatment: Active TB infection should be treated in consultation with an infectious disease provider, but may include the use of isoniazid (INH), pyridoxine, ethambutol, and pyranizamide (24). INH therapy alone is used for LTBI prophylaxis and is recommended for HIV-positive women diagnosed with LTBI in pregnancy.

## Gastroenterology

Differential diagnosis and associated symptoms

1. Gastroenteritis/infectious diarrhea
   a. Associated symptoms: Anorexia, nausea, emesis, malaise, fever, tachycardia, localized versus diffuse abdominal pain, diarrhea
   b. Risk factors: Recent travel to endemic area, sick contacts, improperly prepared or stored food
2. Appendicitis
   a. Associated symptoms: May include right lower quadrant pain (80%) or right upper quadrant pain (10–55%) (25)
   b. Diagnostic workup: Graded compression ultrasonography is the preferred first-line diagnostic test as it avoids ionizing radiation. The sensitivity of ultrasonography is reported as 66–100% with a 95% specificity (26). A noncompressible blind-ending tubular structure with diameter 76 mm supports the diagnosis of appendicitis. The American College of Radiology suggests the use of ultrasonography and magnetic resonance imaging as the most appropriate imaging modalities for working up right lower quadrant pain in pregnancy (27).
   c. Summary: Acute appendicitis is the most common cause of acute abdominal pain in pregnancy, with an estimated incidence of 1:800–1:1500 (25). Pregnancy is associated with a higher rate of appendiceal perforation than in nonpregnant adults (55% versus 4–19%) and may be partially explained by the delay in diagnosis and therapy. The risk of fetal loss is increased in the setting of perforation, peritonitis, or appendiceal abscess (25).
3. Cholecystitis
   a. Associated symptoms: Nausea and emesis. See the associated symptoms for appendicitis.
   b. Risk factors: Cholelithiasis (present in 3.5–10% of pregnant women) (28).
   c. Diagnostic workup: Ultrasound (95–98% sensitivity). Conventional criteria = sonographic Murphy's sign, presence of cholecystolithiasis, gallbladder size of >4 cm, gallbladder sludge, gallbladder wall size of >4 mm, and pericholecystic fluid (28).
   d. Summary: Acute cholecystitis occurs in 1/1600–10,000 pregnancies. Maternal morbidity is the same as for nonpregnant patients and fetal risk cited as 1–2% (28). With a presentation typically identical to nonpregnant patients, however, Murphy's sign is less relevant in advanced gestational age (28).
4. Listeriosis
   a. Associated symptoms: Fever, influenza-like illness, abdominal or back pain, vomiting/diarrhea, headache, myalgia, sore throat, or may present without any symptoms
   b. Risk factors: Travel, consumption of unpasteurized dairy products, sick contacts
   c. Diagnostic workup: Amniotic fluid, blood, and urine cultures
   d. Summary: *L. monocytogenes* is a Gram-variable rod typically transmitted via oral ingestion that may result in mild to severe illness in pregnant women (29). Maternal listeriosis may result in chorioamnionitis, spontaneous abortion, stillbirth, or fetal infection during pregnancy (30). Maternal illness may be mild and self-limited, however, the mortality rate of pregnant patients with Listeria meningitis has been reported as high as 29%, which is higher than the 17% described in nonpregnant adults (17).
   e. Treatment is ampicillin with trimethoprim–sulfamethoxazole being considered second-line therapy for the nonpregnant patient with penicillin allergy.
5. Hepatitis
   a. Associated symptoms: Anorexia, jaundice, fatigue, abdominal pain, nausea and vomiting, diarrhea, dark urine, and pale stools

   b. Risk factors: IV drug use, partner with hepatitis, blood transfusions, needle sharing, high-risk sexual behavior, consumption of contaminated food (especially clams/oysters)

   c. Diagnostic workup: Hepatitis serologies, liver function testing

   d. Summary: Fever is an uncommon presenting symptom for hepatitis; acute hepatitis A is the most likely to present with fever (31). Presentation may be variable; the incubation period is typically 10–50 days, during which transmissibility to others is highest. A prodromal phase may then be seen with the preceding symptoms. The icteric phase generally begins within 10 days of symptom onset, and the fever usually improves after the first few days of jaundice. Hepatitis A is transmitted via the fecal–oral route. The mortality risk is 0.2% in the icteric phase, but a small percentage of patients may clinically worsen and develop fulminant hepatitis, characterized by high fever, severe abdominal pain, jaundice, and hepatic encephalopathy. This phase has an associated mortality of 70–90%.

   e. Postexposure prophylaxis: In the setting of hepatitis A exposure in pregnancy, the immune status should be determined with hepatitis A serological testing followed by immunization and monitoring for symptoms. Treatment is supportive care if symptoms develop.

## Genitourinary

Differential diagnosis and associated symptoms

1. HSV primary versus recurrence
   a. Associated symptoms: Ulcerative genital lesion, influenza-like illness, dysuria, incomplete voiding, back or abdominal pain, lymphadenopathy
   b. Risk factors: Exposure to HSV, high-risk sexual behavior
   c. Diagnostic workup: HSV PCR or culture, serology to determine past exposure history
   d. Summary: Approximately 22% of pregnant women are seropositive for HSV-2. HSV-1 accounts for 15–20% of new anogential lesions in young women (32). A primary HSV-1 or HSV-2 anogenital outbreak carries a 57% risk of neonatal herpes infection (33). A primary infection may present with painful genital ulcers or vesicles, fever, lymphadenopathy, dysuria, or other nonspecific genitourinary symptoms. Patients may also be asymptomatic. HSV hepatitis should be distinguished from HELLP (hemolysis, elevated liver enzymes, low platelet count) syndrome and may similarly present with transaminitis, liver dysfunction, and abdominal pain. Other associated symptoms may include maternal viral sepsis, pneumonitis or encephalitis (34). Disseminated HSV in pregnancy is rare but may carry a 50% mortality rate (35).

2. Acute HIV
   a. Associated symptoms: Influenza-like illness, lymphadenopathy, night sweats, unexplained weight loss
   b. Risk factors: Multiple sexual partners, IV drug use, history of intimate partner violence, incarceration, transactional sex
   c. Diagnostic workup: HIV antibodies, HIV ribonucleic acid PCR (viral load), CD4 T-cell count
   d. Summary: A new diagnosis of HIV in pregnancy warrants referral to a specialist with experience in treating HIV in pregnancy. Antiretroviral (ARV) therapy should be offered to all pregnant women and the choice of ARV is based on viral resistance pattern, medical comorbidities, safety and toxicity profiles of medications, and patient compliance. HIV staging should include the assessment of need for opportunistic infection prophylaxis, TB exposure, and immunization history. Therapy goals are to decrease HIV viral load and increase CD4 counts to decrease the risk of vertical/perinatal transmission. Without any interventions, perinatal transmission is 14–42%, depending on the setting (36).

3. Pyelonephritis
   a. Associated symptoms: Dysuria, costovertebral angle tenderness
   b. Risk factors: Risk factors include asymptomatic bacteriuria, urinary tract infections—these increase risk for pyelonephritis by 20–30% (37). Additional risk factors include urinary tract stones or malformations, diabetes mellitus, multiparity, and low socioeconomic status (38).
   c. Summary: Pyelonephritis affects up to 2% pregnancies and is the most common nonobstetric indication for antepartum hospital admission (38,39). It may be associated with serious sequelae including pneumonia, ARDS, and sepsis (39). Pyelonephritis in pregnancy increases the risk for mechanical ventilation, acute heart failure, pulmonary edema, and acute renal failure (39).

4. Group A streptococcal infection
   a. Associated symptoms: Lower abdominal or perineal pain, vaginal discharge, urinary frequency, and diarrhea may accompany genital tract infection (8). Blanching erythema may suggest streptococcal toxic shock syndrome, seen with group A *S. pyogenes* infection. Intramyometrial gas pockets may be concerning for *Clostridium perfringens*; tissue crepitance and disproportionate pain on physical examination may be concerning for necrotizing fasciitis.
   b. Risk factors: Obstetric risk factors—Prolonged rupture of membranes, repeated vaginal examinations, fetal surgery during pregnancy, illegal abortion, cervical cerclage, retained products of conception, obesity, diabetes mellitus, older maternal age, conservative management of placenta accreta, delivery outside a healthcare facility, sick contacts.

## Infectious Sources for Fever

Differential diagnosis and associated symptoms

1. Chora-amniotic infection or inflammation
   a. Summary: Defined as the inflammation or infection of chorion or amnion and should include the following signs/symptoms: maternal fever (oral temperature of >39°C or 102.2°F at a single time point of two measurements, >38°C or 100.4°F, taken 30 minutes apart) *plus* fetal tachycardia (greater than 160 beats per minute for 10 minutes or longer), maternal white blood cell (WBC) count greater than 15,000 in the absence of corticosteroids, purulent fluid from the cervical os, *or* biochemical or microbiological amniotic fluid results consistent with the microbial invasion of the amniotic cavity. Isolated maternal fever can occur during labor in the setting of epidural anesthesia, hyperthyroidism, use of E2 prostaglandins, dehydration, and excessive ambient heat (40).

2. TORCHES
   a. Summary: TORCH infections include toxoplasmosis, other (syphilis), rubella, cytomegalovirus, and HSV. These may present with fever, cutaneous manifestations, ophthalmologic findings, and neurological involvement such as microcephaly, hydranencephaly, or fetal intracranial calcifications (33). See previous section for HSV.

3. Varicella zoster
   a. Associated symptoms: Fever, vesicular rash, dyspnea
   b. Risk factors: Lack of immunity, sick contact or varicella exposure, smoking
   c. Diagnostic workup: VZV serology should be assessed in the setting of exposure in the absence of prior infection or childhood exposure
   d. Summary: Varicella incidence in pregnancy is estimated to be 1–5 cases per 10,000 pregnancies (41). Disease severity is typically worse among adults and pregnant women. Exposure at 8–20 weeks of pregnancy is associated with an increased risk of congenital varicella. Exposure after 20 weeks or peripartum increases the risk of neonatal varicella.

Nonimmune pregnant patients with exposure should be offered postexposure prophyalxis with varicella immune globulin. Pregnant patients who develop VZV should be treated with acyclovir. Varicella pneumonia complicates 10–20% of VZV cases in pregnancy and may develop within 1 week of rash onset. Prior to antiviral treatment, VZV pneumonitis was associated with a 30–40% mortality rate, with current rates estimated at <15% (41).

4. Postabortal infection

    a. Associated symptoms: Infection following surgical abortion is 0.5% and 0.01–0.21% following medical abortion (9). Clinical signs or symptoms may include any of the following: adnexal tenderness, fever, uterine tenderness, abdominal or pelvic pain, heavy vaginal bleeding, and vaginal discharge. Importantly, only about one-third of women will present with fever (10). The Centers for Disease Control and Prevention definition of pelvic inflammatory disease should be used, which defines the condition with of the following (cervical motion tenderness, uterine tenderness or adnexal tenderness) (11).

    b. Risk factors: Age less than 20 years, presence of chlamydia or bacterial vaginosis, prior history of pelvic inflammatory disease (9).

    c. Diagnostic workup: While a diagnosis of pelvic inflammatory disease can be made clinically, supporting testing can include an elevated erythrocyte sedimentation rate and C-reactive protein, pathologic wet mount, abnormal ultrasound, endometrial biopsy, or laparoscopic findings (9).

    d. Summary: Postabortal infections are a rare complication but should be considered in the patient presenting with cervical motion, uterine, or adnexal tenderness in the setting of recent pregnancy termination.

5. Mosquito-borne illnesses (Zika)

    a. Associated symptoms: A thorough travel history can help establish the appropriate differential diagnosis. Only 20% of individuals affected by Zika will experience symptoms, and these are typically fever, chills, conjunctivitis, rash, and arthritis.

    b. Risk factors: Residence or travel in/to endemic areas, sexual activity with a partner who lives in or has recently travelled to an endemic area.

    c. Diagnostic workup: see Centers for Disease Control and Prevention website for up-to-date testing alogrithms regarding Zika screening in pregnancy.

    d. Summary: Maternal Zika in pregnancy is typically a self-limited illness but can have profound implications for the pregnancy itself. Congenital Zika syndrome is still being described but appears to have the most serious sequelae in the first trimester. Severe microcephaly and other central nervous system abnormalities are the hallmark of this syndrome.

## Other Causes of Fever

1. Epidural: Intrapartum fever ($T > 100.4°F$ or $38°C$) occurred in 14.5% of women receiving epidural anesthesia compared to 1% of women not receiving an epidural (adjusted OR: 14.5; 95% CI: 6.3–33.2). In the presence of maternal epidural, the temperature may rise between 0.08–0.14°C per hour (42–44).

    Fetal management during a febrile episode is shown in Box 12.1.

---

**BOX 12.1   FETAL MANAGEMENT DURING FEBRILE EPISODE**

Fetal tachycardia or tachysystole may be seen in response to maternal fever. Fetal heart rate variability may be decreased, minimal, or absent. The use of tocolytics in the setting of severe maternal illness should be carefully considered, as the use of β-agonists may increase the risk of pulmonary edema. Reducing maternal fever with acetaminophen will help lower the fetal heart rate back to baseline (21).

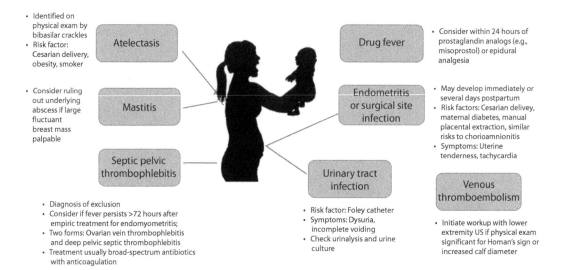

- Identified on physical exam by bibasilar crackles
- Risk factor: Cesarian delivery, obesity, smoker

Atelectasis

Drug fever

- Consider within 24 hours of prostaglandin analogs (e.g., misoprostol) or epidural analgesia

- Consider ruling out underlying abscess if large fluctuant breast mass palpable

Mastitis

Endometritis or surgical site infection

- May develop immediately or several days postpartum
- Risk factors: Cesarian delivey, maternal diabetes, manual placental extraction, similar risks to chorioamnionitis
- Symptoms: Uterine tenderness, tachycardia

Septic pelvic thrombophlebitis

Urinary tract infection

Venous thromboembolism

- Diagnosis of exclusion
- Consider if fever persists >72 hours after empiric treatment for endomyometritis;
- Two forms: Ovarian vein thrombophlebitis and deep pelvic septic thrombophlebitis
- Treatment usually broad-spectrum antibiotics with anticoagulation

- Risk factor: Foley catheter
- Symptoms: Dysuria, incomplete voiding
- Check urinalysis and urine culture

- Initiate workup with lower extremity US if physical exam significant for Homan's sign or increased calf diameter

FIGURE 12.4    Postpartum sources of fever.

## Postpartum Considerations

Differential diagnosis and associated symptoms

1. Atelectasis
2. Infection: Endometritis, surgical site infection
3. Urinary tract infection (cystitis, pyelonephritis)
4. Drug fever
5. Venous thromboembolism
6. Septic pelvic thrombophlebitis
7. Mastitis

Postpartum sources of fever are shown in Figure 12.4.

## REFERENCES

1. Dreier JW, Anderson A-MN, Berg-Beckhoff G. Systematic Review and Meta-analyses: Fever in Pregnancy and Health Impacts in the Offspring. *Pediatrics*. 2014;133(3):e674-e688.
2. Albright CM, Ali TN, Lopes V, Rouse DJ, Anderson BL. The Sepsis in Obstetrics Score: A Model to Identify Risk of Morbidity from Sepsis in Pregnancy. *Am J Obstet Gynecol*. 2014;211(39):e1-e8.
3. Seymour CW, Liu VX, Iwashyna TJ, Brunkhorst FM, Rea TD, Scherag A et al. Assessment of Clinical Criteria for Sepsis: For the Third International Consensus Definitions for Sepsis and Septic Shock (Sepsis-3). *JAMA*. 2016;315(8):762-774.
4. Bauer ME, Bauer ST, Rajala B, MacEachern MP, Polley LS, Childers D et al. Maternal Physiologic Parameters in Relationship to Systemic Inflammatory Response Syndrome Criteria. *Obstet Gynecol*. 2014;124(3):535-541.
5. Singer M, Deutschman CS, Seymour CW, Shankar-Hari M, Annane D, Bauer M et al. The Third International Consensus Definitions for Sepsis and Septic Shock (Sepsis-3). *JAMA*. 2016;315(8):801-810.
6. Shankar-Hari M, Phillips GS, Levy ML, Seymour CW, Liu VX, Deutschman CS et al. Developing a New Definition and Assessing New Clinical Criteria for Septic Shock: For the Third International Consensus Definitions for Sepsis and Septic Shock (Sepsis-3). *JAMA*. 2016;315(8):775-787.

7. Guntupalli KK, Hall N, Karnad DR, Bandi V, Belfort M. Critical Illness in Pregnancy Part I: An Approach to a Pregnant Patient in the ICU and Common Obstetric Disorders. *Chest.* 2015;148(4):1093-1104.

8. Guntupalli KK, Karnad DR, Bandi V, Hall N, Belfort M. Critical Illness in Pregnancy Part II: Common Medical Conditions Complicating Pregnancy and Puerperium. *Chest.* 2015;148(5):1333-1345.

9. Chebbo A, Tan S, Kassis C, Tamura L, Carlson RW. Maternal Sepsis and Septic Shock. *Crit Care Clin.* 2016;32:119-135.

10. Centers for Disease Control and Prevention. Pregnancy Mortality Surveillance System 2016. Available at https://www.cdc.gov/reproductivehealth/maternalinfanthealth/pmss.html.

11. Say L, Chou D, Tuncalp O, Moller A-B, Daniels J, Gulmezoglu AM et al. Global Causes of Maternal Death: A WHO Systematic Analysis. *Lancet Glob Health.* 2014;2:323-333.

12. Ghaffari N, Dossett E, Lee RH, Paola A. Antipsychotics Leading to Neuroleptic Malignant Syndrome in Pregnancy. *Obstet Gynecol.* 2012;119:436-438.

13. Berman BD. Neuroleptic Malignant Syndrome: A Review for Neurohospitalists. *The Neurohospitalist.* 2011;1(1):41-47.

14. De Leo S, Lee SY, Braverman LE. Hyperthyroidism. *Lancet.* 2016;388:906-918.

15. de Veciana M. Diabetic ketoacidosis in pregnancy. *Seminars in Perinatology.* 2013;37:267-273.

16. Landrum LM, Hawkins A, Goodman JR. Pneumococcal Meningitis during Pregnancy: A Case Report and Review of Literature. *Inf Dis Obstet Gynecol.* 2007:1-3.

17. Adriani KS, Brouwer MC, van der Ende A, van de Beek D. Bacterial Meningitis in Pregnancy: Report of Six Cases and Review of the Literature. *Clin Microbiol Infect.* 2012;18:345-351.

18. Schoen C, Kischkies L, Elias J, Ampattu BJ. Metabolism and Virulence in Neisseria meningitidis. *Front Cell Infect Microbiol.* 2014;4:114.

19. Cox S, Hankins G, Leveno K, Cunningham F. Bacterial Endocarditis: A Serious Pregnancy Complication. *J Reprod Med.* 1988;33:671-674.

20. Shah M, Patnaik S, Wongrakpanich S, Alhamshari Y, Alnabelsi T. Infective Endocarditis due to Bacillus cereus in a Pregnant Female: A Case Report and Literature Review. *IDCases.* 2015;2(3):120-123.

21. Barton JR, Sibai BM. Severe Sepsis and Septic Shock in Pregnancy. *Obstet Gynecol.* 2012;120(3):689-706.

22. Sheffield JS, Cunningham FG. Community-Acquired Pneumonia in Pregnancy. *Obstet Gynecol.* 2009;114(4):915-922.

23. Malhame I, Cormier M, Sugarman J, Schwartzman K. Latent Tuberculosis in Pregnancy: A Systematic Review. *PloS One.* 2016;11(5):e0154825.

24. Birsner M, Graham EM. Cardiopulmonary Disorders of Pregnancy. In: Hurt JK, Guile MW, Bienstock JL, Fox HE, Wallach EE, editors. *The Johns Hopkins Manual of Gynecology and Obstetrics*, 4th ed. Philadelphia, PA: Lippincott Williams & Wilkins; 2011. pp. 195-207.

25. Kelly TF, Savides TJ. Gastrointestinal Disease in Pregnancy. In: Creasy R, Resnik R, Iams JD, Lockwood CJ, Moore TR, Greene MF, editors. *Creasy and Resnik's Maternal-Fetal Medicine: Principles and Practice*, 7th ed. Elsevier Saunders; 2014, pp. 1059-1074.

26. Williams R, Shaw J. Ultrasound Scanning in the Diagnosis of Acute Appendicitis in Pregnancy. *Emerg Med J.* 2007;24:359-360.

27. Rosen M, Ding A, Blake M, Baker M, Cash B, Fidler J et al. ACR Appropriateness Criteria Right Lower Quadrant Pain-Suspected Appendicitis. *J Am Coll Radiol.* 2011;8(11):749-755.

28. Bouyou J, Gaujoux L, Marcellin M, Leconte F, Goffinet C, Chapron C et al. Abdominal Emergencies during Pregnancy. *J Visc Surg.* 2015;152(6):S105-S115.

29. Mylonakis E, Paliou M, Hohmann EL, Calderwood SB, Wing EJ. Listeriosis during pregnancy: A Case Series and Review of 222 Cases. *Medicine.* 2002;81(4):260-269.

30. Jackson KA, Iwamoto M, Swerdlow D. Pregnancy-associated Listeriosis. *Epidemiol. Infect.* 2010;138(10):1503-1509.

31. World Health Organization. Hepatitis A. *Fact Sheets* 2017; http://www.who.int/mediacentre/factsheets/fs328/en/.

32. Workowski KA, Bolan GA. Sexually Transmitted Diseases Treatment Guidelines, 2015. MMWR Recommendations and reports/ Centers for Disease Control. 2015;64(Rr-03):1-137.

33. Stephenson-Famy A, Gardella C. Herpes Simplex Virus Infection during Pregnancy. *Obstet Gynecol Clin N Am.* 2014;41:601-614.

34. Brown Z, Gardella C, Wald A. Genital Herpes Complicating Pregnancy. *Obstet Gynecol.* 2005;106:845-856.

35. Anzivino E, Fioreti D, Mischitelli M, Bellizzi A, Barucca V, Chiarini F et al. Herpes Simplex Virus Infection in Pregnancy and in Neonate: Status of Art of Epidemiology, Diagnosis, Therapy and Prevention. *Virol J.* 2009;6(40):1-11.

36. Eppes C, Anderson J. HIV in Pregnancy. In: Hurt JK, Guile MW, Bienstock JL, Fox HE, Wallach EE, editors. *The Johns Hopkins Manual of Gynecology and Obstetrics*, 4th ed. Philadelphia, PA: Lippincott Williams & Wilkins; 2011. pp. 186-194.

37. Glaser AP, Schaeffer AJ. Urinary Tract Infection and Bacteriuria in Pregnancy. *Urol Clin N Am.* 2015;42:547-560.

38. Wing D, Fassett M, Getahun D. Acute Pyelonephritis in Pregnancy: An 18-year Retrospective Analysis. *Am J Obstet Gynecol.* 2014;210(219):1-6.

39. Dotters-Katz S, Heine RP, Grotegut CA. Medical and Infectious Complications Associated with Pyelonephritis among Pregnant Women at Delivery. *Infect Dis Obstet Gynecol.* 2013;2013(124102):1-6.

40. Higgins R, Saade G, Polin R, Grobman W, Buhimschi I, Watterberg K et al. Evaluation and Management of Women and Newborns with a Maternal Diagnosis of Chorioamnionitis: Summary of a Workshop. *Obstet Gynecol.* 2016;127(3):426-436.

41. Gnann JW. Varicella-Zoster Virus: Prevention Through Vaccination. *Clin Obstet Gynecol.* 2012;55(2):560-570.

42. Lieberman E, Lang JM, Frigoletto Jr F, Richardson DK, Ringer SA, Cohen A. Epidural Analgesia, Intrapartum Fever, and Neonatal Sepsis Evaluation. *Pediatrics.* 1997;99:415-419.

43. Fusi L, Maresh M, Steer P, Beard R. Maternal Pyrexia Associated with the Use of Epidural Analgesia in Labour. *Lancet.* 1989;333(8649):1250-1252.

44. Vinson D, Thomas R, Kiser T. Association between Epidural Analgesia during Labor and Fever. *J Fam Pract.* 1993;36(6):617-622.

# 13

## Obstetric Hemorrhage I: Antepartum Hemorrhage

**John C. Smulian, MD, MPH, Casey Brown, DO, and Amanda Flicker, MD**

## CONTENTS

## Overview

First trimester bleeding occurs in over 20% of pregnancies (1). First trimester hemorrhage makes up only a small portion of cases of first trimester bleeding, although the exact incidence of early true hemorrhage is unknown. Significant obstetric bleeding after the first trimester and prior to labor is less common, but is usually clinically significant. History, physical examination, laboratory studies, and ultrasound aid in making the diagnosis. The differential diagnosis for antepartum hemorrhage regardless of trimester includes a heterogeneous group of etiologies (Table 13.1). The approach to management should be targeted to the gestational age and specific etiology with careful attention to the needs of both the mother and the fetus. However, many of the principles of management are the same, regardless of the gestational age or etiology, which is optimal for the standardization of management and creates opportunities for simulation training.

## Maternal History and Physical Examination

The initial approach to the assessment and management of the mother is similar across trimesters (Tables 13.2 and 13.3). Obtaining a good obstetric history is critical, but should not delay the implementation of standard measures to ensure the cardiovascular and pulmonary stability of the mother. Targeted history features that can direct the establishment of an etiology in later pregnancy are listed in

TABLE 13.1

Differential Diagnosis for the Most Common Etiologies of Antepartum Hemorrhage

- First trimester etiologies
  - Abortion (threatened, inevitable, incomplete)
  - Cervical ectopic pregnancy
  - Cesarean scar pregnancy
  - Other ectopic pregnancy
  - Cervical polyp or lesion
  - Trauma/lacerations
  - Arteriovenous malformations
  - Molar pregnancy
- Second/third trimester etiologies
  - Placenta previa
  - Placental abruption
  - Vasa previa
  - Uterine rupture
  - Lacerations
  - Medical conditions
  - Miscellaneous

TABLE 13.2

Targeted History Can Guide the Direction of Interventions

- Gestational age
- Recent trauma
- Antecedent coitus
- History of prior uterine surgery
- History of substance abuse
- Medical conditions that might be associated with an increased bleeding risk (platelet or coagulation disorders)
- Details of previous episodes of bleeding in the pregnancy
- Bleeding characteristics (onset timing, amount, and duration)
- Symptoms suggestive of cardiovascular instability such as syncope, dizziness, palpitations, anxiety, and nausea
- Symptoms of abdominal, pelvic, or vaginal pain may also be helpful
- Prior ultrasound findings that can be associated with placental bleeding or abruption (pregnancy of unknown location, subchorionic hematoma, molar gestation, placenta previa, low placenta, vasa previa, mullerian abnormalities of the uterus, or fibroids)
- Second trimester- and third trimester-specific history
  - History of a prior abruption
  - Hypertensive disorders (chronic hypertension or preeclampsia)
  - Symptoms suggestive of undiagnosed preeclampsia (headache, scotomata, epigastric pain, malaise, significant recent weight gain, or edema)

Table 13.4. These measures include the assessment and stabilization of the ABCs (airway, breathing and circulation). The determination of whether antenatal bleeding is clinically significant must be quickly performed and often lacks precision. The proportion of maternal cardiac output directed toward the uterus increases by approximately 6 to 12% as a pregnancy approaches term, which increases the risk for catastrophic hemorrhage (2). Therefore, it is reasonable to approach the care of women presenting with more than "spotting" as if there is a potential for significant hemorrhage, especially if the pregnancy is at a gestational age of potential fetal viability. Fortunately, most episodes of bleeding in pregnancy are self-limited and spontaneously resolve.

Signs that may indicate clinically significant hemorrhage include maternal tachycardia (>100 beats per minute [bpm] or >10% increase over the baseline), hypotension (<100 mmHg systolic or <60 mmHg diastolic), dyspnea, diaphoresis, agitation, or other mental status changes and pallor. Occasionally, bradycardia can be encountered with significant blood loss (3). Blood noted on clothing or on the maternal legs and feet is highly suggestive of significant hemorrhage. The estimation of the amount of blood loss based on the number of pads used or blood in the toilet can be unreliable. The gynecologic literature has demonstrated much variability in self-estimates of blood loss with gynecologic bleeding (4). There are

TABLE 13.3

Targeted Physical Examination Elements

- Vital signs
  - Maternal tachycardia often precedes hypotension in obstetric hemorrhage. (Normal maternal heart rate range in pregnancy is 80–110 bpm)
  - Bradycardia with severe hemorrhage
  - Hypotension
  - Elevated blood pressures of >140 mmHg systolic or >90 mmHg diastolic may indicate preeclampsia after 20 weeks, which is a risk factor for placental abruption
  - Tachypnea
- Pallor
- Agitation or altered mental status
- Abdominal tenderness or rebound in upper abdomen
- Vaginal examination by speculum (observe for polyps/masses, cervicitis, lacerations, varicosities, cervical dilation, fetal parts)
- Cervical examination in the first trimester for dilation and pregnancy tissue
- Cervical examination in the second or third trimester is contraindicated until there is confirmation that there is no placenta previa—either from a prior ultrasound examination or one at the time of presentation
- Uterine tenderness (often seen with abruption or infection)
- Uterine tonus (persistent contraction often seen with abruption)
- Confirm fetal cardiac activity

TABLE 13.4

Targeted Second or Third Trimester History Information with Possible Associated Hemorrhage Etiologies

| History | Hemorrhage Etiology |
|---|---|
| Early pregnancy bleeding | Placenta previa |
| | Low-lying placenta |
| | Vasa previa |
| | Abruption |
| Prior abruption | Abruption (10–20% recurrence rate) |
| Placental implantation abnormalities on ultrasound | Placenta previa |
| | Low-lying placenta |
| | Vasa previa |
| | Abruption |
| Mullerian abnormality | Abruption |
| Fibroids (especially if >6 cm) | Abruption |
| Hypertensive disorders | Abruption |
| Trauma | Abruption (abdominal trauma) |
| | Lacerations (vaginal trauma) |
| Recent coitus | Vaginal or cervical lacerations |
| Prior uterine surgery | Uterine rupture |
| Platelet and coagulation abnormalities | Exacerbates bleeding from all other etiologies |
| Substance abuse (e.g., cocaine and amphetamines) | Abruption |
| Abdominal pain | Abruption |
| | Traumatic abdominal injury |
| | Uterine rupture |
| | Labor |
| No abdominal pain | Placenta previa |
| | Low-lying placenta |
| | Vasa previa |
| | Lacerations |
| | Varicosities |
| Vaginal pain | Lacerations |
| | Varicosities |

TABLE 13.5

Clinical Signs of Hypovolemia

| Amount of Blood Loss | Clinical Signs |
|---|---|
| 1000 mL | Slight change in blood pressure, heart rate normal, palpitations, respiratory rate normal, dizziness, normal urine output |
| 1500 mL | Narrowed pulse pressure, heart rate over 100, respiratory rate is 20–30, diaphoretic, weak, urine output is 20–30 mL/hour |
| 2000 mL | Hypotension, narrowed pulse pressure, heart rate over 120, respiratory rate is 30–40, pale, extremities cool, restlessness, urine output is 5–15 mL/hour |
| ≥2500 mL | Profound hypotension, heart rate over 140, respiratory rate over 40, slight urine output or anuria |

*Source:* Used from David Lagrew, MD, Audrey Lyndon, RNC, CNS, PhD, Elliott Main, MD, Larry Shields, MD, Kathryn Melsop, MS, Debra Bingham, RN, Dr. PH. Obstetric Hemorrhage Toolkit: Improving Health Care Response to Obstetric Hemorrhage. (California Maternal Quality Care Collaborative Toolkit to Transform Maternity Care) Developed under contract #08-85012 with the CDPH/MCAH Division; Published by the California Maternal Quality Care Collaborative, June 2010.

several classifications of hemorrhage severity. One useful tool is presented in Table 13.5 (5). It is important to remember that hemorrhage severity classifications should be treated as guidelines since they generally have not been accurately validated prospectively for pregnancy. Another important point is that physiological changes are a continuum and individual responses to hemorrhage may vary based on a variety of individual factors such as age, body mass index, gestational age, and comorbidities. Therefore, rigid adherence to classification systems to judge severity and to determine management should not be a substitute for good clinical judgment and situational awareness. Nevertheless, they can be a very helpful adjunct to assist with communication among the multiple team members involved in the acute care of these women and to judge the need for transfusion, clinical deterioration, or improvement.

## Laboratory Testing

Laboratory tests useful for the assessment and management of antepartum hemorrhage include the following:

- Beta human chorionic gonadotropin (HCG) in first trimester
- Complete blood count (± differential based on infection suspicion)
- Comprehensive metabolic profile
  - Electrolytes, renal and hepatic function
- Coagulation profile (prothrombin time, partial thromboplastin time, fibrinogen)
- Blood type and crossmatch for blood products
  - O-negative blood may be most readily available
  - Alert for possible need for fresh frozen plasma, cryoprecipitate, and platelets
- Drug screen
- Urine protein/creatinine ratio and uric acid (if preeclampsia is suspected)

## Fetal Assessment

The initial approach to the evaluation and care for acute antepartum hemorrhage should always be focused on the stabilization and care of the mother. However, there are a number of fetal considerations that are important and can help with decision-making, especially with regard to delivery. It is critical to establish the gestational age of the pregnancy as part of the initial evaluation, since decisions about delivery are dependent on the potential for fetal survival. Ideally, this should come directly from a read-ily accessible medical record, but can also be determined from the patient, family members, or others on site with specific knowledge of the pregnancy. A clinical assessment of the uterine size can also give information about gestational age, but can be misleading in the presence of growth restriction, rupture of membranes, multiple gestation, and concealed hemorrhage (abruption). Generally, in singleton preg-nancies, the top of the uterus is at the pelvic brim around 12 weeks and at the level of the umbilicus at 20 weeks. The distance of the fundus from the umbilicus increases by 1 cm for each week of gestation thereafter. Ultrasound can be used to accurately assess gestational age, but performance of an ultrasound should not delay the initiation of measures to stabilize the mother.

Continuous fetal heart rate (FHR) monitoring with the assessment of contractions with tocodynamom-etry is the best way to assess the immediate fetal condition after ≥24 weeks. This requires the presence of fetal monitoring equipment. If the patient is evaluated in an emergency room setting, a fetal monitor should be obtained from the labor and delivery suite. In the absence of electronic monitoring, intermittent auscultation can be used, but the effectiveness in the setting of active obstetric bleeding is not established.

Abnormal monitoring patterns that should prompt consideration for delivery include the following:

- Sustained baseline fetal tachycardia of >160 bpm
- A sinusoidal FHR pattern (persistent sine-wave pattern with a cycle frequency of 3–5 per minutes)
- Periodic FHR decelerations
- Absent or minimal variability
- Prolonged decelerations (sustained FHR of ≤15 bpm for ≥2 but <10 minutes)
- Frequent spontaneous uterine contractions (>5 per 10 minutes over at least 30 minutes)

## Ultrasound

Ultrasound can be used in several ways to assist with the evaluation and management of antenatal hemor-rhage. It may be helpful for the establishment or confirmation of gestational age, determination of pla-cental location, assessment of abruption, evaluation of fetal well-being, and evaluation of fetal anemia. Its role in evaluating a suspected uterine rupture is not clear.

### First Trimester Assessment

The pregnancy location should be established if not done previously. The most common life-threatening cause of first-trimester hemorrhage is an ectopic pregnancy. While these are usually located in the fal-lopian tubes, pregnancy implantations can occasionally implant in the cervix or in the niche created by the scar in the lower uterine segment from a prior cesarean delivery (Figure 13.1). The presence of a yolk sac or fetal pole within a gestational sac in the uterus is a reliable predictor of an intrauterine pregnancy (IUP). The most common sign of an adnexal ectopic pregnancy on ultrasound is an adnexal mass. Other ultrasonography findings suggestive (not diagnostic) of an ectopic pregnancy are beta HCG level of >2000 mIU without an IUP seen on transvaginal ultrasound, echogenic or complex free peritoneal fluid (indicating blood), and a "tubal ring," which is a fluid-filled center and trophoblastic tissue as the outer ring (6). However, clinicians must be cautious in using beta HCG discriminatory levels for diagnosing an ectopic pregnancy since normal IUPs can occur even if not visualized with levels of >2000 mIU (7). A molar pregnancy has an ultrasound appearance that has been described as a "snowstorm" (Figure 13.1).

### Gestational Age Assessment

In the first trimester, the gestational age is best established by a crown rump length measurement. Later in pregnancy, a transcerebellar diameter is the best single measurement to assess the gestational age (±3 days). This requires some degree of advanced ultrasound expertise (8). A rapid assessment of the

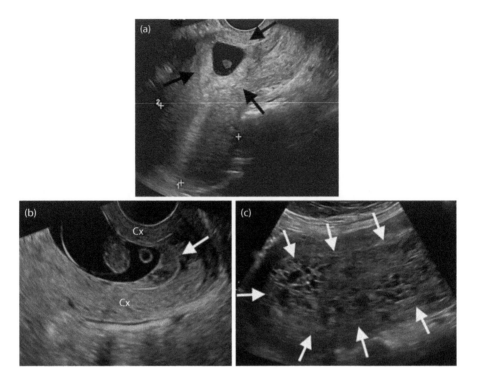

**FIGURE 13.1**   Ultrasound image of abnormal early gestation implantations: (a) cesarean scar pregnancy within the niche of a prior lower uterine segment cesarean scar (*black arrows*), an empty upper uterus, and closed cervix (Cx); (b) cervical ectopic (*white arrows*) with intact pregnancy distending the endocervical canal (Cx indicates anterior and posterior cervix); and (c) a molar pregnancy with a snowstorm appearance (*white arrows*).

gestational age using only a femur length can estimate the gestational age within 2 weeks and is easier to obtain. The use of multiple biometry measurements that include the biparietal diameter, abdominal circumference, and femur length can confirm the gestational age with greater confidence and can be used to estimate the fetal weight, although these measurements can take time to obtain (Figure 13.2) (9).

## Placental Assessment in the Second or Third Trimester

If a prior ultrasound determined that the lower edge of the placenta was >2 cm from the internal os, then significant bleeding from a low placental implantation is unlikely (10,11). However, a prior ultrasound that showed a placenta previa, a low-lying placenta, or a vasa previa suggests that placental or fetal vessel bleeding would be the most likely etiology of the hemorrhage. It is essential to confirm the placental location prior to performing a digital cervical examination, since the manual disruption of a placenta previa can lead to catastrophic bleeding. Importantly, even if a prior placenta previa has resolved, there may still be a residual vasa previa that can spontaneously rupture, usually after 34 weeks (12). Bleeding from a vasa previa is an obstetric emergency and requires urgent delivery for fetal indications, even though the maternal condition is usually unaffected. Ultrasounds for placental location and for vasa previa not only are highly accurate when transvaginally performed, but can also be performed with a translabial approach with an abdominal transducer covered by a sterile glove (Figure 13.3). Although the diagnosis is often straightforward using color Doppler imaging when the vessels are intact, the accuracy of detection in the presence of a bleeding vessel is not known.

Ultrasound can be used to identify placental abruption, although accuracy rates are considered low (13). Sonographic features may include a preplacental chorionic plate hematoma; subplacental hematoma; placental implantation displacement; subchorionic hematoma/fluid collection; placental parynchemal hemorrhage, which "wiggles" when stimulated with a transducer bounce; and intraamniotic debris.

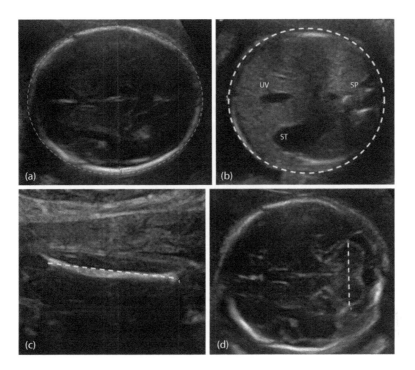

FIGURE 13.2   Ultrasound biometry examples useful for estimating gestational age and weight: (a) biparietal diameter and head circumference; (b) abdominal circumference with landmarks (umbilical vein [UV], stomach [ST], spine [SP]); (c) femur length; and (d) transcerebellar diameter.

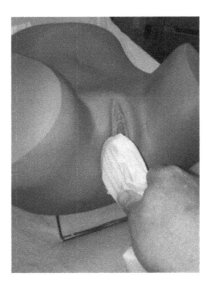

FIGURE 13.3   Simulated approach to translabial ultrasound to assess for placenta previa when transvaginal imaging is not available. Place sterile glove over transabdominal probe prior to scanning.

Ultrasound-identified abruptions are clinically significant, and delivery should be considered in the presence of active hemorrhage. If abruption is suspected, it is important to assess the mother for PEC, which is a significant risk factor. PEC should be strongly considered with elevated blood pressures, headaches, visual changes, epigastric or right upper quadrant pain, low platelets, elevated liver enzymes, and a urine protein/creatinine ratio of ≥0.3 (14).

## Fetal Condition Assessment

The ultrasound assessment of fetal well-being is important in the management of antepartum obstetric hemorrhage after 24 weeks, particularly if the mother is stabilized and expectant management is considered.

- Biophysical profile (BPP): If the FHR monitor shows minimal or absent variability, absent accelerations, decelerations, or baseline tachycardia, a BPP (the assessment of fetal movement, tone, fluid volume, breathing and the nonstress test) can be performed to determine whether there is a fetal indication for delivery. A persistent BPP of ≤6/10 can be considered for delivery when the mother is stabilized, but each case should be individualized based on gestational age, as well as available resources for maternal and infant care.
- Fetal Doppler: Abruption can be associated with fetal anemia and can be assessed with the pulse Doppler interrogation of the middle cerebral artery (15). Elevations of the peak systolic velocity (≥1.5 multiples of the median) are associated with significant fetal anemia and may be used for an indication for delivery at gestational ages at or near term. In situations when a fetal transfusion is not appropriate (unstable bleeding) or in the presence of an unstable placenta (15).
- Fetal growth restriction: The presence of an estimated fetal weight of <5th percentile for the gestational age may indicate a fetus with less reserve that is more vulnerable to injury. Delivery in this situation can be considered, especially after 34 weeks of gestation.

## Management

The severity and etiology of the hemorrhage, along with the gestational age, are the primary determinants of management. The primary initial goal is always the stabilization of the mother, followed by assessment of the fetus for possible delivery. Reasonable approaches to the management of antepartum bleeding based on gestational age and common etiologies are described in Table 13.6 and algorithms

TABLE 13.6

Primary Treatment Modalities for Significant Hemorrhage by Suspected Etiology

| *First Trimester* | |
|---|---|
| Abortion | Uterine evacuation |
| Ectopic–adnexal | Surgical treatment |
| Ectopic–cervical | Surgical treatment/uterine artery embolization/balloon tamponade |
| Ectopic–cesarean scar | Surgical treatment/uterine artery embolization/balloon tamponade |
| Cervical polyp | Ligation and/or removal |
| Trauma/lacerations | Surgical repair |
| Arteriovenous malformation | Embolization/surgical treatment |
| Molar pregnancy | Uterine evacuation |
| | |
| *Second or Third Trimester*[a] | |
| Placenta previa | Delivery if ≥34 weeks/individualize care if <34 weeks |
| Placental abruption | Delivery if ≥34 weeks/individualize care if <34 weeks |
| Vasa previa | Delivery if ≥24 weeks |
| Uterine rupture | Delivery emergently |
| Lacerations | Surgical repair |
| Medical conditions | Condition-specific treatment |
| Varicosities | Compression/surgical repair |

[a] Consider use of steroids (two doses of betamethasone 12 mg IM 24 hours apart) to promote fetal maturity if preterm (24–36 weeks) and clinical status allows.

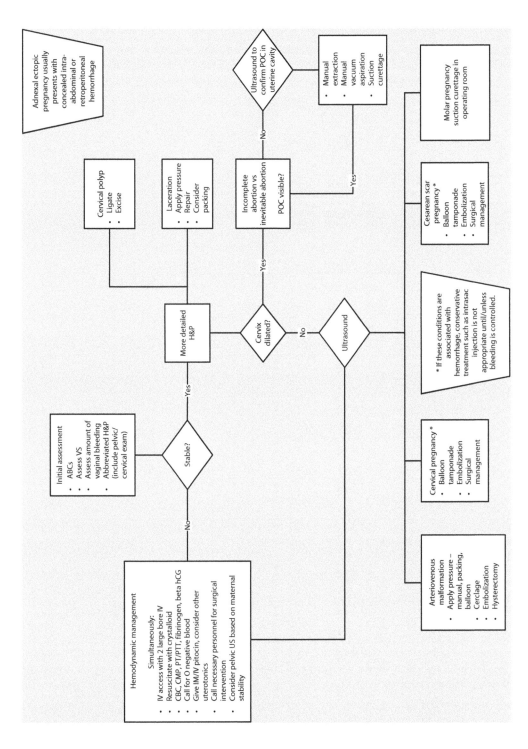

**FIGURE 13.4**  Flowchart for the evaluation and management of early pregnancy hemorrhage.

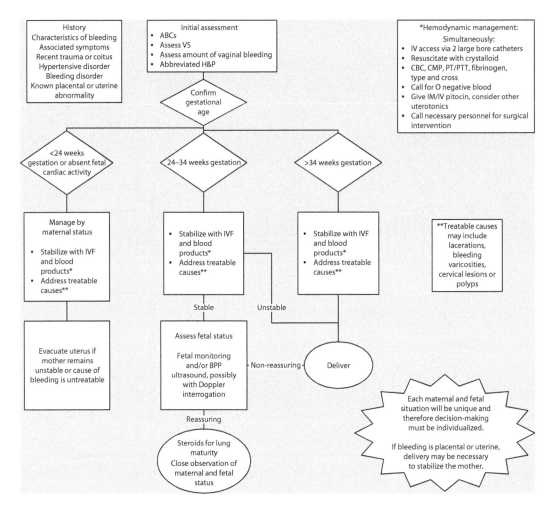

FIGURE 13.5    Flowchart for the evaluation and management of antepartum hemorrhage in the second and third trimesters.

are shown in Figures 13.4 and 13.5. While algorithms cannot cover all situations, they can be useful for guiding the overall approach to care.

## Considerations for Management of First-Trimester Hemorrhage

### General Principles

- Assess vital signs including oxygenation status
- Establish airway and ventilation if compromised
- Establish intravenous (IV) access
- Administer oxygen
- Assess amount of vaginal bleeding
- Obtain targeted history
- Perform a targeted physical examination
  - Abdominal examination

- Pelvic and cervical exam
  - If products of conception are palpable or visible, they can be removed bedside, which can stop hemorrhage

## Special Considerations if Stable

When the patient is stable and there is access to ultrasound imaging, proceed with an abdominal and pelvic ultrasound as a next step in order to help differentiate between hemorrhage from an intrauterine pregnancy with an abortion (threatened, inevitable, or incomplete); a cesarean scar implantation; a cervical ectopic; and a molar pregnancy; since the management differs based on the diagnosis.

- Genital lacerations of the labia, vagina, or cervix are usually due to traumatic injury, but are not always associated with sexual assault. If assault is suspected, then follow applicable laws and procedures for the evaluation and collection of evidence. Good visualization of the entire lower genital tract is required during examination to assess the location and extent and often requires anesthesia for optimal exposure.
- Cervical polyps rarely cause hemorrhage. However, large ones prolapsed through the external cervical os can usually be clamped for tamponade and either high ligated or removed.
- A dilated cervix in conjunction with products of conception (POCs) on ultrasonography is either an inevitable abortion or an incomplete abortion. Both are treated with the removal of the POCs.
  - If POCs are visible on exam, they can often be removed during the initial pelvic examination. Afterward, the ultrasound should be performed an empty uterus.
  - If POCs are not visible on exam, and one has access to a manual vacuum aspirator (MVA), this is a procedure that may be performed bedside to remove the POCs up until 12 weeks of gestation (16). If the MVA is not available, one should proceed with going to the operating room for a vacuum curettage.
- If the cervix is not dilated and an ultrasound shows an intrauterine pregnancy, the diagnosis is based on the potential viability of the pregnancy. A nonviable pregnancy is considered a missed abortion. The features of a nonviable pregnancy are noted in Table 13.7 (7).
  - In this situation, a dilatation and evacuation procedure using an MVA or vacuum curettage is indicated.
  - If the pregnancy is confirmed as viable, then the clinician must decide whether the patient is stable enough to expectantly manage, with hopes of preserving the pregnancy, or whether to proceed with emptying the uterus. If there is any concern that the mother is not stable, then maternal health should take precedence and the uterus should be emptied.
- If an unrecognized cesarean scar pregnancy or cervical ectopic is treated with dilation and evacuation, there may be extensive hemorrhage. If either is identified and the patient is stable, then consult with experienced clinicians for additional management that might include intrasac injection of KCl or methotrexate, surgical resection, or balloon compression with a double balloon catheter (17,18). If this is suspected during a curettage procedure, hemorrhage may be temporarily controlled until more definitive treatment is available, by clamping the length of

## TABLE 13.7

Diagnostics of a Nonviable Pregnancy[a]

- Crown-rump length of ≥7 mm and no cardiac activity
- Mean gestational sac diameter of ≥25 mm and no embryo
- Absence of an embryo with cardiac activity ≥14 days after a scan that showed a gestational sac without a yolk sac
- Absence of an embryo with cardiac activity ≥11 days after a scan that showed a gestational sac with a yolk sac

*Source:* Doubilet, P. M. et al., *New England Journal of Medicine*, 369, 1443–1451, 2013.

[a] A pregnancy that cannot result in a live-born baby and includes failed intrauterine pregnancies and ectopic implantations.

TABLE 13.8

Commonly Used Uterotonic Medications and Dosing Regimen

| Agent | Dose | Route | Frequency | Contraindications |
|-------|------|-------|-----------|-------------------|
| Oxytocin | 10–40 units in 500–1000 mL crystalloid | IV (alternate 10 units IM) | Continuous (≤80 units) | None |
| Methylergonovine | 0.2 mg | IM | Every 2–4 hours | Hypertensive disorders |
| Misoprostol | 800–1000 mcg | PR (alternate PO) | One time | None |
| Prostaglandin F2 alpha | 0.25 mg | IM (alternate intramyometrial) | Every 15–90 minutes up to eight doses | Pulmonary, cardiac, renal, or hepatic disease |
| Prostaglandin E2 | 20 mg | PR | Every 2 hours | Hypotension |

*Note:*  IM, intramuscular; IV, intravenous; PR, per rectum; PO, per os (oral).

the endocervical canal at 3:00 and 9:00 with an instrument such as a pair of ringed forceps or by utilizing a balloon tamponade with a 24 French catheter with a 30–60 cm³ balloon.

- If a molar pregnancy is suspected, then a vacuum curettage is indicated, preferably with ultrasound guidance and the availability of blood for transfusion.

Consider the following maneuvers to control bleeding that is persistent after uterine evacuation:

- Bimanual compression or massage
- Uterotonics (Table 13.8)
- Consider a Foley balloon tamponade in the first trimester
- In a stable patient
  - Uterine artery embolization if available
- In an unstable patient
  - Possible exploratory laparotomy with adjunct procedures:
    1. Uterine artery ligation (fertility sparing)
    2. Uterine compression sutures (fertility sparing)
    3. Uterine packing (fertility sparing)
    4. Hysterectomy
- When the bleeding resolves or significantly decreases, continue to give IV pitocin for at least the next 1–2 L of fluid infusion at a concentration of 10–20 units pitocin/L
- Confirm Rh status and administer Rh immunoglobin injection for Rh-negative unsensitized women

## Considerations for the Management of Second- and Third-Trimester Hemorrhage

### General Principles

- Assess vital signs including oxygenation status
- Establish airway and ventilation if compromised
- Establish IV access
- Administer oxygen
- Assess amount of vaginal bleeding
- Obtain targeted history
- Perform a targeted physical examination

- Abdominal examination
- Speculum examination should be gentle to avoid cervical disruption and to allow the examination of the lower genital tract for bleeding lacerations or cervical problems
- Manual cervical exam *only if no placenta previa and the inferior placental margin is known to be >2 cm from the internal os*
- Be prepared for possible postpartum hemorrhage if delivery is performed

## Special Considerations if Stable

- Genital lacerations of the labia, vagina, or cervix and cervical polyps should be managed the same as in the first trimester (see previous section).
- Place on continuous FHR monitoring with contraction monitoring.
- If the patient is stable and there is access to ultrasound imaging, proceed with imaging to help evaluate the etiology and guide management.
- Treat any underlying medical conditions such as coagulation disorders, and stop any medications that would interfere with coagulation hemostasis (heparin and its derivatives, aspirin, etc.).
- If ≥37 weeks, consider delivery in controlled circumstances.
- If <37 weeks,
  - Betamethasone: 12 mg intramuscular (IM), two doses, 24 hours apart for the promotion of fetal maturity (24–36 6/7 weeks)
  - Tocolysis is usually contraindicated if active preterm labor with hemorrhage
  - Consider delivery for progressive preterm labor, recurrent hemorrhage or maternal deterioration, and suspected fetal compromise (abnormal FHR pattern, abnormal BPP, or suspected fetal anemia)
  - If no immediate indication for delivery, hospitalization with expectant monitoring and daily fetal assessment is recommended. The duration of hospitalization and plan of care should be individualized in consultation with experts in complicated pregnancy management such as maternal–fetal medicine specialists.
- Can consider vaginal delivery in very selected circumstances with stable mother and fetus, no ongoing hemorrhage, evidence of spontaneous labor progress, and no evidence of placenta or vasa previa.

While the majority of antepartum episodes of significant hemorrhage will resolve after the uterus is emptied regardless of trimester, on occasion, there may be persistent bleeding after uterine evacuation or delivery. For evaluation and assessment in this situation, refer to Chapter 14.

## REFERENCES

1. Sapra KJ, Buck Louis GM, Sundaram R, Joseph KS, Bates LM, Galea S et al. Signs and symptoms associated with early pregnancy loss: Findings from a population-based preconception cohort. *Hum Reprod.* 2016; 31:887-896.
2. Flo K, Wilsgaard T, Vårtun A, Acharya G. A longitudinal study of the relationship between maternal cardiac output measured by impedance cardiography and uterine artery blood flow in the second half of pregnancy. *BJOG.* 2010; 117:837-844.
3. Kirkman E, Watts S. Haemodynamic changes in trauma. *Br J Anaesth.* 2014; 113:266-275.
4. Pai M, Chan A, Barr R. How I manage heavy menstrual bleeding. *Br J Haematol.* 2013; 162:721-729.
5. Lagrew D, Lyndon A, Main E, Shields L, Melsop K, Bingham D. Obstetric Hemorrhage Toolkit: Improving Health Care Response to Obstetric Hemorrhage. (California Maternal Quality Care Collaborative Toolkit to Transform Maternity Care) Developed under contract #08-85012 with the CDPH/MCAH Division; Published by the California Maternal Quality Care Collaborative, June 2010.
6. Kirk E. Ultrasound in the diagnosis of ectopic pregnancy. *Clin Obstet Gynecol.* 2012; 55:395-401.

7. Doubilet PM, Benson CB, Bourne T, Blaivas M, Society of Radiologists in Ultrasound Multispecialty Panel on Early First Trimester Diagnosis of Miscarriage and Exclusion of a Viable Intrauterine Pregnancy, Barnhart KT et al. Diagnostic criteria for nonviable pregnancy early in the first trimester. *N Engl J Med.* 2013; 369:1443-1451.

8. Chavez MR, Ananth CV, Smulian JC, Yeo L, Oyelese Y, Vintzileos AM. Fetal transcerebellar diameter measurement with particular emphasis in the third trimester: A reliable predictor of gestational age. *Am J Obstet Gynecol.* 2004; 191:979-984.

9. Hadlock FP, Harrist RB, Carpenter RJ, Deter RL, Park SK. Sonographic estimation of fetal weight: The value of femur length in addition to head and abdomen measurements. *Radiology.* 1984; 150:535-540.

10. Vintzileos AM, Ananth CV, Smulian JC. Using ultrasound in the clinical management of placental implantation abnormalities. *Am J Obstet Gynecol.* 2015; 213:S70-S77.

11. Oyelese Y, Smulian JC. Placenta previa, placenta accreta, and vasa previa. *Obstet Gynecol.* 2006; 107(4):927-441.

12. Oyelese Y, Catanzarite V, Prefumo F, Lashley S, Schachter M, Tovbin Y et al. Vasa previa: The impact of prenatal diagnosis on outcomes. *Obstet Gynecol.* 2004; 103:937-942.

13. Oyelese Y, Ananth CV. Placental abruption. *Obstet Gynecol.* 2006; 108:1005-1016.

14. Gillon TE, Pels A, von Dadelszen P, MacDonell K, Magee LA. Hypertensive disorders of pregnancy: A systematic review of international clinical practice guidelines. *PLoS One.* 2014; 9:e113715.

15. Society for Maternal-Fetal Medicine, Mari G, Norton ME, Stone J, Berghella V, Sciscione AC et al. Society for Maternal-Fetal Medicine (SMFM) Clinical Guideline #8: The fetus at risk for anemia—Diagnosis and management. *Am J Obstet Gynecol.* 2015; 212:697-710.

16. Kinariwala M, Quinley KE, Datner EM, Schreiber CA. Manual vacuum aspiration in the emergency department for management of early pregnancy failure. *Am J Emerg Med.* 2013; 31(1):244-247.

17. Timor-Tritsch IE, Monteagudo A, Bennett TA, Foley C, Ramos J, Kaelin Agten A. A new minimally invasive treatment for cesarean scar pregnancy and cervical pregnancy. *Am J Obstet Gynecol.* 2016; 215:351.e1-e8.

18. Timor-Tritsch IE, Monteagudo A. Unforeseen consequences of the increasing rate of cesarean deliveries: Early placenta accreta and cesarean scar pregnancy—A review. *Am J Obstet Gynecol.* 2012; 207:14-29.

# 14

## Obstetric Hemorrhage II: Postpartum Hemorrhage

**Amanda Flicker, MD, Casey Brown, DO, and John C. Smulian, MD, MPH**

**CONTENTS**

## Introduction

Postpartum hemorrhage (PPH) has been variously defined as excessive bleeding occurring in the first 24 hours after delivery, estimated blood loss of ≥500 mL after vaginal delivery and ≥1000 mL after cesarean, bleeding associated with a hematocrit drop of 10 percentage points, and need for transfusion and hemodynamic instability (1). Recent efforts to consolidate definitions have led to an American College of Obstetricians and Gynecologists-endorsed hemorrhage definition of cumulative blood loss of ≥1000 mL or blood loss accompanied by sign/symptoms of hypovolemia within 24 hours following the birth process (includes intrapartum loss) (2). All can reasonably be used to identify clinically significant postpartum bleeding. PPH complicates up to 6% of all deliveries and remains one of the leading causes of maternal morbidity and mortality globally (1,3,4).

The management of PPH includes two primary components: (a) identifying and controlling the cause of the bleeding and (b) assessing and stabilizing the hemodynamic status of the patient. Anticipation and preparedness are critical components in the management of this life-threatening condition. PPH can be preceded by antepartum hemorrhage; see Chapter 13. Antepartum hemorrhage from placenta previa and placental abruption can continue, even after delivery. Although there are risk factors that can be identified both antepartum and intrapartum to help clinicians anticipate hemorrhage (Table 14.1), unfortunately,

TABLE 14.1

Common Antepartum and Intrapartum Risk Factors for Postpartum Hemorrhage

| Antepartum | Intrapartum | Postpartum |
|---|---|---|
| Uterine fibroids (large, numerous, and/or obstructing) | Chorioamnionitis | Operative vaginal delivery |
| Multiple gestation | Prolonged labor | Cesarean birth (unplanned) |
| >4 prior vaginal births | Prolonged or high-dose oxytocin use | Retained placenta |
| Chorioamnionitis | Ongoing active bleeding | Extensive lacerations |
| Prior postpartum hemorrhage | Magnesium sulfate prophylaxis | |
| Prior uterine surgery including cesarean | Prolonged second stage | |
| Abnormal placentation (previa, accreta, abruption) | | |
| Anemia with other risk factors | | |
| Thrombocytopenia | | |
| Active bleeding (>bloody show) | | |
| Coagulopathy, i.e., Von Willebrand's disease | | |

PPH often occurs in women without identifiable risk factors and can be life threatening. Therefore, all delivery units and providers should be prepared to respond to this true obstetric emergency.

## Anticipation, Systems, and Planning

### Antenatal Care

The correction of preexisting anemia in at-risk pregnancies is important and should be aggressively pursued (5). Multidisciplinary planning for patients at the highest risk, i.e., suspected invasive placental disease, can also be highly effective in reducing maternal morbidity and mortality (6).

### Admission Risk Assessment

Completing a hemorrhage risk assessment for every patient on admission for delivery can promote situational awareness as well as lead to appropriate anticipatory actions for the safety of the patient. Ongoing assessments in labor and at delivery should also be completed at regular intervals (7,8), and changes in risk status should be communicated to the entire team.

## Preparedness

Considering that the blood supply to the placenta at term is as much as 600 mL/minute and the average circulating blood volume is approximately 6 L, it may take only 10 minutes for the entire blood volume to pass through the uterus (9). For this reason, hemorrhage in the postpartum setting can be swift and catastrophic. It is essential that all birthing units are prepared to quickly respond with appropriate medications, equipment, personnel, and blood products. All providers should be prepared to implement a stepwise medical and surgical approach to manage PPH and its causes.

Although every delivery has the potential to be complicated by PPH, the incidence can be reduced using a variety of simple measures. The active management of the third stage of labor (AMTSL) is an evidence-based approach for the prevention of PPH. Components include the following:

1. Prophylactic administration of an uterotonic agent before delivery of the placenta (oxytocin preferred)
2. Controlled traction of the umbilical cord after cord clamping and transaction

Randomized trials suggest that the uterotonic agent is the most important component of AMTSL and can reduce postpartum blood loss (10). The value of aggressive uterine massage may be less than has been historically assumed.

## Supplies and Medications

Having prepared supplies and medications readily available in the delivery unit facilitates more rapid and efficient response to a PPH. This avoids treatment delays that are inevitable when needed items must be requested from a central supply area. Every birthing unit should organize supplies to facilitate accessibility during hemorrhage emergencies. As with any medications or sterile items, regular inspection is recommended to assess expiration dates and facilitate restocking.

It is generally recommended that all delivery units have an *obstetric hemorrhage emergency cart*, well stocked with equipment and supplies commonly used to manage PPH (Table 14.2). A portable *obstetric hemorrhage medication box* can be used to store the most commonly used uterotonic medications. These medications should be available through verbal orders and administered using closed-loop communication. Having to obtain access for each medication separately in a pharmacy storage unit or from a pharmacy located far from the delivery unit can dangerously delay treatment. Syringes and needles to administer the medications can be kept with the medication box or in the obstetric emergency cart. A simple table should be affixed to the box to remind providers of safe dosing practices for the various medications used in these emergent situations (Table 14.3).

## Protocol and Policy Development

Emergency care protocols and policies are vitally important to ensure consistent response during the evolution of a PPH. Examples are the following.

### Obstetric Rapid Response Team (OB RRT)

Delivering institutions should have a predetermined and readily available team to be activated when there is initial recognition of a PPH. The members of the team may vary based upon the available resources for the delivery setting, but may include obstetricians (attending and/or resident), anesthesia providers, and the charge nurse. It is important to specify an institution-specific communication process for how the team will be summoned, such as by burst page, overhead call, or simple phone tree. A simple message such as "OB RRT to room # for hemorrhage" can be sent and participants can receive brief report on arrival to the bedside.

TABLE 14.2

Examples of Selected Contents of an Obstetric Hemorrhage Emergency Cart

- IV start: Large bore angiocatheters, IV tubing, saline/LR, IV pressure bags
- Blood draw tubes: Complete blood count (CBC), blood chemistry, coagulation studies, type and cross—banded together in bundles for ease of use
- Foley catheters with urimeter bags
- Uterine tamponade balloon with instructions for use and fluid for instillation
- Suture for B-Lynch (or maintain in OR labeled for that use) with diagram
- Diagram for uterine artery ligation
- Hunter's (banjo) curette
- Consider equipment for vaginal laceration management
  Suture (variety of sizes and maternals)
  Retractors (right angle, Deaver, Breisky, and Gelpi)
  Vaginal packing

*Note:* IV, intravenous; LR, lactated ringers; OR, operating room.

TABLE 14.3

Commonly Used Pharmacological Uterotonic Interventions for Use during a Postpartum Hemorrhage

| Agent | Dose | Route | Frequency | Contraindications |
|---|---|---|---|---|
| Oxytocin | 10–40 units in 500–1000 mL crystalloid | IV (alternate 10 units IM) | Continuous to a maximum of 80 units | None |
| Methylergonovine | 0.2 mg | IM | Every 2–4 hours | Hypertensive disorders |
| Misoprostol | 800–1000 mcg | PR (alternate PO) | One time | None |
| Prostaglandin F2 alpha | 0.25 mg | IM (alternate intramyometrial) | Every 15–90 minutes to a maximum of eight doses | Pulmonary, cardiac, renal, or hepatic disease |
| Prostaglandin E2 | 20 mg | PR | Every 2 hours | Hypotension |

*Note:*   IM, intramuscular; IV, intravenous; PO, per os (oral); PR, per rectum.

## Obstetric Hemorrhage Protocol

If the initial rapid response does not control the hemorrhage (see the "Management" section), the team response should escalate. Many institutions treat this situation as a hospital emergency by announcing an obstetric emergency, such as a "Code Crimson." This triggers the notification of additional services such as the blood bank, laboratory, critical care unit, and nursing supervisor. In addition, the chain of communication should specify the activation and notification of other providers needed to support escalation in care. The specific individuals identified will depend on the institution or setting-specific resources, but may include additional obstetric surgeons, a gynecologic oncologist, a trauma or general surgeon, or a perfusionist for cell saver technology. It is important that the individuals involved in these teams recognize that a substantial portion of these Code Crimson events ultimately will not require actual participation of all potential team members. Nevertheless, all team members should respond when the protocol is activated due to the unpredictable course of an individual event.

## Massive Transfusion Protocol

Every institution providing obstetric care should have a plan to respond to a need for high-volume blood transfusions (11). Many institutions initiate a *massive transfusion protocol* early in the management of obstetric-related hemorrhage to avoid delays in administration of blood products. This plan can be initiated after giving two to four units of packed red blood cells (RBCs) when there is continued heavy bleeding, with vital signs changes in the setting of uncontrolled bleeding, with suspected coagulopathy, or when the hemorrhage is anticipated to be massive, as in the setting of invasive placental disease (also known as placenta accreta or morbidly adherent placenta). Most obstetric massive transfusion protocols have been adapted from the nonpregnancy trauma experience and have not been prospectively validated. All protocols include interventions such as adequate intravenous (IV) access, volume expansion, uterotonics, and blood replacement therapy. Many also include the use of tranexamic acid, although there are limited data on optimum use in acute PPH. The routine use of recombinant factor VIIa in obstetric hemorrhage is not recommended due to the lack of effect on mortality and variable effect on morbidity in nonobstetric populations. However, institution-specific guidelines for use can be considered under circumstances of severe hemorrhage unresponsive to other therapies. Table 14.4 contains some suggested components of a massive transfusion protocol.

## Transfer Policies and Plans

It is important to have a plan for transfer to a tertiary care facility when a PPH occurs in a facility where resources are limited. Clear lines of communication should be delineated with the receiving facility to

**TABLE 14.4**

Components of a Massive Transfusion Protocol

- Activate with suspected blood loss of 30–40% and/or hemodynamic changes. Should have already received two units of packed RBCs and 2 L of IV fluid
- Notification of the blood bank and activation of communication chain, including runners and scribes
- Request multiple blood product units to be released together, typically four to six units of packed RBCs, fresh frozen plasma and pooled platelet packs
- Can use O-negative blood until cross-matched product is available
- Use high-flow warming infuser if available
- Transfuse a standard ratio of packed RBCs and fresh frozen plasma with platelet packs (e.g., a ratio of 1:1:1 to 3:2:2)
- Administer fibrinogen concentrates such as cryoprecipitate (5–10 units) after 6–8 units of FFP or if fibrinogen level is <100 mg/dL
- Tranexamic acid can be used as supplemental treatment to prevent fibrinolysis (1 g over 10 minutes as loading dose then 1 g infusion over next 8 hours)

provide for an efficient and seamless process that will avoid delays in care. The timing for transfer will be situation specific and will depend on hospital resources, geography, and the stability of patient for transport (12).

## Recognition

The clinical diagnosis of PPH commonly relies on clinical judgment, which is variable and often inaccurate. Providers can overestimate losses, which not only can lead to unnecessary treatment, but can also underestimate losses that are higher than average, leading to delays in vital treatments (13). Visual analog systems are more useful. An example used in our unit is shown in Figure 14.1. Another way to assess blood loss volume is quantitative blood loss (QBL). QBL uses weights and measures to assess blood loss, usually at the time of delivery, while subtracting other fluid volumes that can interfere with more precise measurement. While QBL is not perfect, it is considered more accurate than simple blood loss estimation by clinicians (14).

- Measure blood loss using a calibrated drape for vaginal birth or a suction canister for cesarean birth.
- Blood loss = volume after placenta – volume before placenta (allows exclusion of amniotic fluid from the assessment of blood loss).
- Subtract any fluids used for irrigation.
- Weigh soaked sponges, pads, underbuttock pads.
  - Blood loss = soaked product – dry weight (1 g = 1 mL).

Blood loss assessment tools should be used to guide interventions such as blood product administration and mobilization of additional resources (see Figure 14.2; see Lagrew et al. (8)). Blood product and coagulation component interventions useful for the management of replacement therapy are found in Table 14.5.

## Management

In order to adequately treat PPH, an etiology-specific management should be considered for primary PPH that occurs within <24 hours of delivery. The most common causes are related to the 4Ts (tone, tissue, trauma, and thrombin). Management should be focused on treating the primary cause(s). A general approach to assessing and managing PPH is provided in an algorithm format in Figure 14.3.

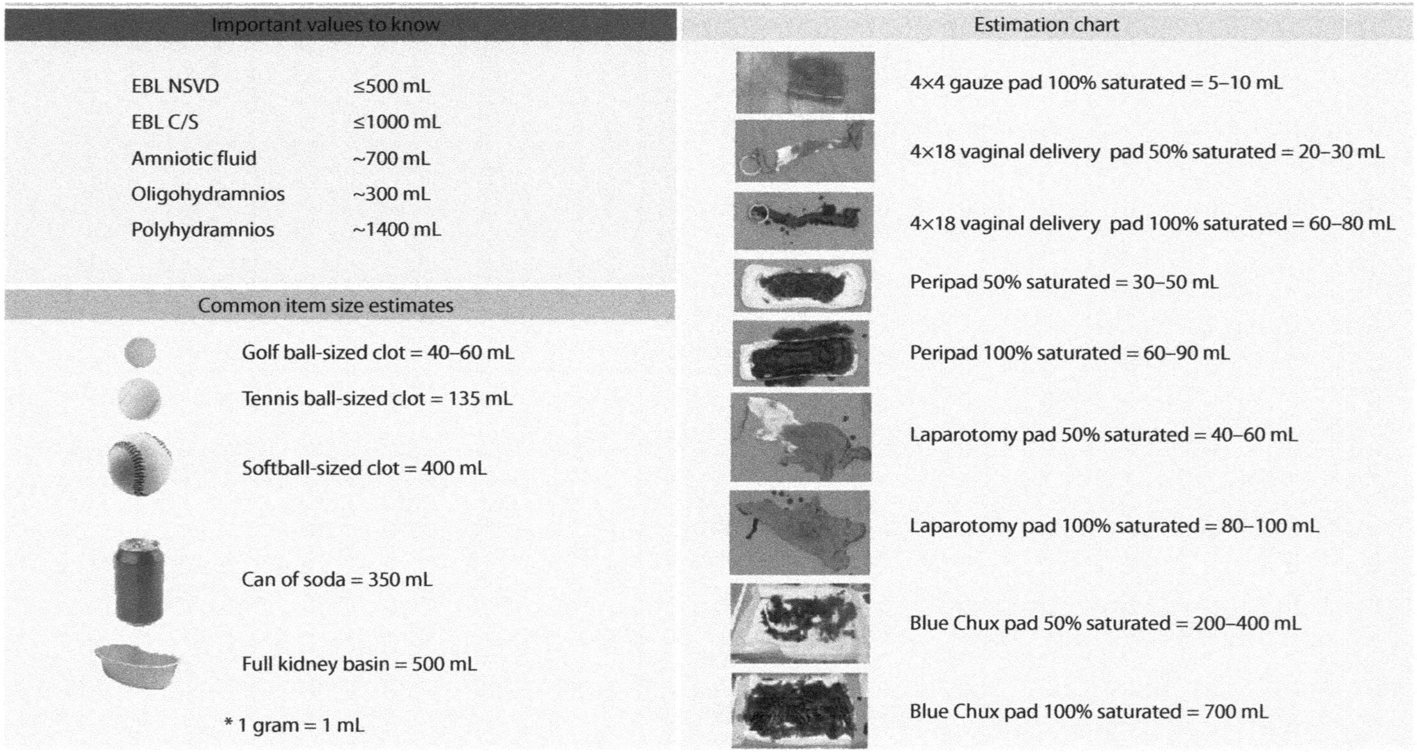

| Important values to know | |
|---|---|
| EBL NSVD | ≤500 mL |
| EBL C/S | ≤1000 mL |
| Amniotic fluid | ~700 mL |
| Oligohydramnios | ~300 mL |
| Polyhydramnios | ~1400 mL |

**Common item size estimates**

Golf ball-sized clot = 40–60 mL

Tennis ball-sized clot = 135 mL

Softball-sized clot = 400 mL

Can of soda = 350 mL

Full kidney basin = 500 mL

* 1 gram = 1 mL

**Estimation chart**

4×4 gauze pad 100% saturated = 5–10 mL

4×18 vaginal delivery pad 50% saturated = 20–30 mL

4×18 vaginal delivery pad 100% saturated = 60–80 mL

Peripad 50% saturated = 30–50 mL

Peripad 100% saturated = 60–90 mL

Laparotomy pad 50% saturated = 40–60 mL

Laparotomy pad 100% saturated = 80–100 mL

Blue Chux pad 50% saturated = 200–400 mL

Blue Chux pad 100% saturated = 700 mL

**FIGURE 14.1** Visual analogue poster to assist with quantifying obstetric blood loss and recognition of obstetric hemorrhage. (Courtesy of Lehigh Valley Health Network, Lehigh County, PA.)

| | Emergency Activation | Physician | Nursing | Other Services |
|---|---|---|---|---|
| **Stage 0**<br>ALL PATIENTS | Assess risk factors | Fundal massage for 15 seconds after delivery of placenta | Oxytocin administration (IV/IM) | |
| **Stage 1—MOBILIZE**<br>>500 mL SVD<br>>1000 mL Cesarean | Mobilize team | Empty bladder<br>Identify etiology of hemorrhage | Large bore IV access<br>IVF resuscitation<br>VS, O₂ sats, cumulative blood loss every 15 min<br>Supplemental O₂<br>Draw labs – CBC, metabolic panel, coagulation studies, type and cross | Additional nursing including charge nurse and physician support<br>Notify anesthesia team |
| **Stage 2—MANAGE**<br><1500 mL<br>Ongoing bleeding<br>VS instability | Activate obstetric hemorrhage protocol | Diagnose and treat etiology of hemorrhage<br>Consider move to OR | Second large bore IV<br>Begin transfusion of pRBC based on clinical signs, not labs<br>Labs every 30–60 min | Blood bank<br>Anesthesia team<br>Additional surgeons<br>Consider trauma team or RRT |
| **Stage 3—MASSIVE**<br>>1500 mL<br>Ongoing bleeding<br>VS instability<br>Blood transfusion<br>Suspicion of DIC | Activate massive transfusion protocol with FFP and platelets after giving 2–4 units pRBC | Move to OR | Upper body warming blanket<br>Apply sequential compression stocking<br>Continue frequent VS, QBL, labs | Critical care team<br>Family support |

FIGURE 14.2  Staged response to obstetric hemorrhage. EBL, estimated blood loss; FFP, fresh frozen plasma; OR, operating room; SVD, spontaneous vaginal delivery.

TABLE 14.5

Blood Product Components and Interventions Useful for Management of Replacement Therapy

| Product | Volume (mL) | Important Contents | Effect |
|---|---|---|---|
| Whole blood | 500 | RBC, plasma, fibrinogen, volume | Increases hematocrit by 3–4% and hemoglobin by 1 g per unit; restores volume and fibrinogen |
| Packed RBCs | 250–300 | RBC with white blood cell (WBC) and platelets; volume | Increases hematocrit by 3–4% and hemoglobin by 1 g per unit |
| Platelets | 50 | Platelets with RBC; WBC and platelets | 5000 per unit, use 6–10 units or single-donor apheresis unit raises platelet count by 30,000 |
| Fresh frozen plasma | 250 | Fibrinogen with all clotting factors including V, VIII, and antithrombin III; volume | Increases fibrinogen to 10 mg/dL; restores volume |
| Cryoprecipitate | 15–50 | Fibrinogen and selected other clotting factors (VIII and XIII and Von Willebrand factor) | Increases fibrinogen by 10 mg/dL; use in pooled packs of five |

## Tone

Uterine atony accounts for up to 80% of cases of PPH (1). Employ simple steps first. Empty the bladder, perform bimanual uterine massage, and perform manual evacuation of clots and assessment of cavity. Using a sponge over the fingertips may provide an effective and rapid manual curettage to remove retained fragments of placenta and membranes. The use of uterotonic agents in a sequential fashion should not be delayed. Common agents used are described in Table 14.3.

If uterine atony continues, several additional approaches can be entertained. An intrauterine tamponade balloon, specifically designed for control of PPH, can be inserted after either a vaginal delivery

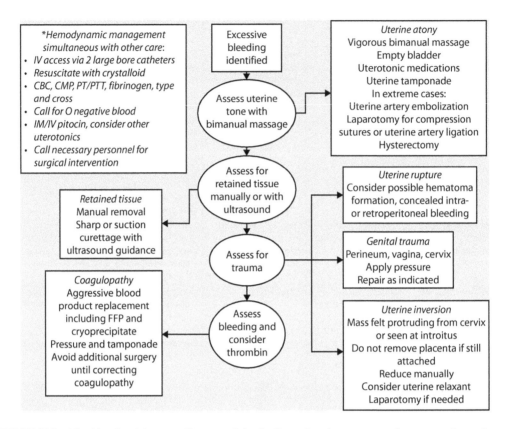

**FIGURE 14.3**   Algorithm for etiology-specific approach for the diagnosis and management of postpartum hemorrhage.

or cesarean. These balloons typically allow inflation with up to 500 mL of crystalloid fluid in order to provide the compression of the uterine lining and are removed 12–24 hours after control of the bleeding. Multiple Foley catheter balloons can be used, but may be less effective due to the size of the uterine cavity in a postpartum uterus. Uterine packing with gauze or surgical laparotomy pads can be used in an emergency, if balloons are not available. A modified "umbrella" pack can be an option: laparotomy pads are placed into a sterile plastic bag, which is snugly pushed into the uterine cavity, with the opening of the bag passing through the cervix into the vagina for later sequential removal of sponges from the bag and then the bag itself. Emergent uterine artery embolization can be considered in hemodynamically stable patients who have not had an adequate response to conservative interventions. Not all institutions will have the radiological expertise for this option.

If the preceding measures have not worked after a vaginal delivery or if there is severe atony with a cesarean, then a surgical approach to the uterus through a laparotomy incision should be considered. Any suspected coagulopathy should be concurrently corrected. Compression sutures are an excellent first step.

The B-Lynch uterine compression suture (Figure 14.4) is considered highly effective at controlling persistent uterine bleeding from atony, although it is not the only uterine compression technique (15,16). It is helpful to have suture intended for uterine compression labeled for its use in each obstetric operating room (OR). It should be a long length and composed of a delayed absorbable material with a large taper needle. Uterine artery ligation as described below can reduce the pulse pressure of blood flow to the uterus to allow time for uterotonic medications and other interventions to work (17).

- The uterus is elevated.
- Tapered needle with delayed absorbable suture is passed anterior to posterior through the myometrium near the isthmus (inferior to the transverse hysterotomy if cesarean).

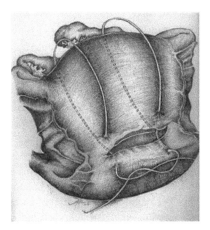

FIGURE 14.4    Schematic of a B-Lynch uterine compression suture. (Courtesy of Anita Sargent, MD.)

- The suture is returned back through an avascular segment of the broad ligament posterior to anterior.
- The suture is tied in order to ligate, but not transect, the ascending branches of the uterine artery.

## Tissue

Retained products of conception can contribute to PPH. Placental inspection should be performed at every delivery to ensure that it is intact with no missing cotyledons. Special care should be taken where placental abnormalities are known, such as a succenturiate lobe or a velamentous cord insertion. If retained placental tissue is suspected, an ultrasound can be utilized to look for retained placental tissue, which is echogenic and heterogeneous (Figure 14.5). When retained placental tissue is suspected, the attendant can evacuate the uterus using manual or surgical techniques. A manual placental removal often can be performed quickly and efficiently after adequate analgesia. Wrapping a gauze sponge around one or two fingers can facilitate the removal of smaller tissue fragments from the uterine cavity. If this is not successful, the possibility of an invasive placenta should be considered. Surgical

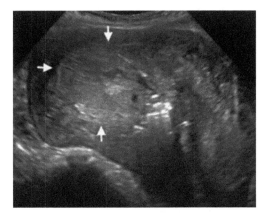

FIGURE 14.5    Ultrasound image of a postpartum uterus with retained placental tissue that is thick and heterogeneous in appearance.

evacuation can be accomplished with a careful sharp curettage (Hunter/banjo curette) or a vacuum curettage. The use of a larger #14 or #16 curved vacurette and large suction tubing are preferred to facilitate the removal of larger tissue fragments. Ultrasound guidance is useful with both manual and surgical evacuation procedures to guide the operator, to reduce the risk of perforation, and to confirm an empty uterus.

## Trauma

The perineum, vagina, and cervix should be carefully examined for bleeding lacerations if the uterus has good tone and no retained products of conception are suspected. In many delivery situations, the visualization of these areas can be a problem. If good lighting, adequate analgesia, proper exposure, and suction are not available in the delivery room, the patient should be moved to an OR. Access to appropriate instrumentation is important. For perineal and lower vaginal lacerations, the use of retractors such as the Gelpi can aid in visibility, especially when assistants are not readily available. For vaginal and deep sulcal lacerations, the use of the Breisky, Deaver, right angle, or other similar tissue retractors will aid with visibility (Figure 14.6). To rapidly inspect for cervical lacerations, one hand depresses the posterior vaginal wall and ring forceps are used to pull the cervix into the field of view while an assistant gives downward fundal pressure to facilitate the cervical descent for adequate visualization. Cervical lacerations require repair if they are bleeding. Packing after repair can help tamponade the laceration for additional approximation and hemostasis. However, all packing material should be tracked to avoid retained foreign bodies. Antibiotics such as a third generation cephalosporin should be administered for the repair of fourth degree lacerations.

## Uterine Inversion

A uterine inversion is considered an obstetric emergency. Prompt identification is paramount. A partially inverted uterus may be felt as a mass through the cervix and into the vagina. A complete uterine inversion usually presents as a mass projecting through the introitus (Figure 14.7). In both situations, the uterine fundus is not palpated in its usual infraumbilical location. The placenta may still be attached and should be left in place until the inversion is rectified, as massive bleeding can ensue from the inability of the surrounding myometrium to contract. Uterine inversion can be erroneously diagnosed as a prolapsed fibroid as it may have similar appearance and feel. This mistake can lead to delayed intervention.

The initial correction of uterine inversion may be accomplished through manual replacement. A cupped hand or a fist can be used to apply pressure to the exposed inverted uterine fundus to replace it

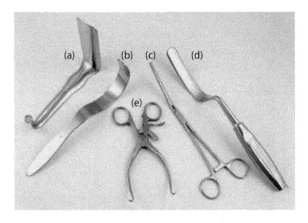

**FIGURE 14.6** Examples of various instruments useful for the management and control of postpartum hemorrhage: (a) right angle retractor, (b) Deaver retractor, (c) Glassman clamp, (d) Breisky retractor, and (e) Gelpi retractor. (Courtesy of Sklar Corporation, West Chester, PA.)

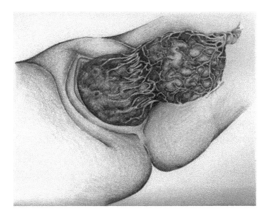

FIGURE 14.7    Schematic of an inverted uterus with placenta immediately after delivery. (Courtesy of Anita Sargent, MD.)

into its anatomic location. Uterine relaxation may be needed and can be achieved using 100–200 mcg (or one to two sprays) nitroglycerin sublingual q2–3 min. Other tocolytics such as terbutaline or magnesium sulfate have been used if nitroglycerin is not available. However, terbutaline can cause tachycardia, which may be misinterpreted as deteriorating hemodynamic status due to hemorrhage. General anesthesia can also be used to relax the uterus. Once the uterus is replaced, uterotonic medications should be used to keep the uterus contracted. Laparotomy is a final option with techniques such as Huntington and Haultain procedures. The Huntington procedure involves the use of Babcock or Allis forceps to elevate the inverted corpus in a progressive and stepwise fashion (18). The Haultain procedure requires an incision in the posterior aspect of the cervical ring and then the elevation of the inverted corpus through that space, followed by closure of the posterior hysterotomy (19). These may also require uterine relaxation to allow inversion correction.

## Uterine Rupture

In the setting of uterine rupture, bleeding can be vaginal, or it can be concealed in the intraperitoneal or retroperitoneal spaces. It should always be considered not only in any patient with risk factors such as prior uterine surgery, prior myomectomy, collagen disorders (classic Ehlers–Danlos syndrome, etc.), or grand multiparity, but also in other patients with unexplained heavy uterine bleeding postpartum or hemodynamic signs such as hypotension and tachycardia. Emergent cesarean delivery and repair of the rupture must occur promptly. Rupture and/or hemorrhage can extend into the broad ligament and retroperitoneal space. The bladder and ureters can be injured in either the rupture or the repair if the rupture extends laterally and caudad. In order to visualize the extent of the laceration, one can place large atraumatic, noncrushing clamps, such as the Glassman clamps, on the edges of the bleeding myometrium in order to minimize the bleeding that can obscure the surgeon's view (see Figure 14.6). Similarly one can rapidly place a running interlocking suture along the medial edge of a laceration that extends down toward the cervix in order to decrease bleeding from this edge, which can improve visualization for optimal repair. Traction on that suture can be used to identify and expose the apex of the laceration to facilitate repair. In some cases, hysterectomy may be the only recourse for catastrophic uterine rupture.

## Thrombin (Coagulopathy)

Clinically significant coagulopathies are important to recognize as contributors to PPH. It is important to identify preexisting coagulation defects such as thrombocytopenia disorders, platelet function abnormalities, Von Willebrand disease, the hemophilias, and other factor deficiencies. Many of these are known prior to pregnancy. Treatment for these disorders should target the underlying disorder (20).

TABLE 14.6

Laboratory Evaluations Helpful in the Management of Acute Obstetric Hemorrhage and DIC

Initial laboratory studies
- Type and cross with antibody screen
- CBC
- Metabolic profile (basic and/or comprehensive)
  Electrolytes
  BUN and creatinine
  Ionized calcium
- Coagulation studies
  Prothrombin time (PT) and international normalized ratio (INR)
  Partial thromboplastin time (PTT)
  Fibrinogen

Repeat labs with ongoing hemorrhage and coagulopathy
- CBC
- Potassium and ionized calcium
- Coagulation studies

There are acquired coagulopathic conditions such as disseminated intravascular coagulopathy (DIC), which is not only most commonly due to hemorrhage, but can also develop after a large placental abruption, sepsis, severe preeclampsia, and amniotic fluid embolism. Importantly, DIC is initially a clinical diagnosis based on various observations of diffuse bleeding from previously hemostatic sites, from venipuncture sites and from other surfaces. Laboratory studies can help confirm the diagnosis, but waiting for results should not delay interventions (Table 14.6). A rapid bedside assessment of a coagulation abnormality can be performed using an extra red top tube of blood that is set aside. Nonclotting of the blood in 8–10 minutes suggests delayed clot formation suggesting a coagulation abnormality. When DIC is suspected, blood and coagulation product replacement should begin immediately and aggressively with the activation of a massive transfusion protocol (Table 14.4). The use of tranexamic acid as an antifibrinolytic therapy may reduce maternal mortality from obstetric hemorrhage when used early if initial medical interventions have failed (21,22).

## Refusal of Blood Products

A unique and challenging situation occurs for patients who decline blood products. These can present clinical, professional, ethical, and legal dilemmas that can be extremely difficult for the patient and the care team. Institutional policies should be developed for the management of these complex cases to provide guidance for care that will avoid the challenges of decision-making under high-stress circumstances. These cases will benefit from informed consent and multidisciplinary team planning. The following are some considerations to maximize good outcomes:

- Optimize antenatal hematocrit
- Determine and document the managements the patient is willing to accept during antenatal care and verify on admission for delivery
- Avoid or mitigate risk factors that are avoidable
- Active management of the third stage of labor
- Aggressive use of uterotonics, surgical techniques, and mobilization of team to avoid DIC
- Cell salvage techniques should be discussed and planned if appropriate
- Use alternate products such as albumin to support blood pressure
- Consider prophylactic or early use of tranexamic acid

# REFERENCES

1. Oyelese Y, Ananth CV. Postpartum hemorrhage: Epidemiology, risk factors, and causes. *Clin Obstet Gynecol*. 2010; 53:147-156.
2. https://www.acog.org/-/media/Departments/Patient-Safety-and-Quality-Improvement/2014reVITALize ObstetricDataDefinitionsV10.pdf?dmc=1&ts=20170713T2118018384; 2017 [accessed July 13, 2017].
3. Quiñones JN, Uxer JB, Gogle J, Scorza WE, Smulian JC. Clinical evaluation during postpartum hemorrhage. *Clin Obstet Gynecol*. 2010; 53:157-164.
4. Ananth CV, Smulian JC. Epidemiology of critical illness in obstetrics. In: Belfort MA, Dildy GA, Saade GR, Phelan JP, Hankins GD, Clark SL, editors. *Critical care obstetrics*. 6th ed. Hoboken, NJ: Blackwell Science; 2017.
5. Anemia in pregnancy: ACOG Practice Bulletin No. 95. American College of Obstetricians and Gynecologists. *Obstet Gynecol*. 2008 (reaffirmed 2017); 112:201-207.
6. Smulian JC, Pascual AL, Hesham H, Qureshey E, Bijoy Thomas M, Depuy AM et al. Invasive placental disease: The impact of a multi-disciplinary team approach to management. *J Matern Fetal Neonatal Med*. 2017; 30:1423-1427.
7. Fleischer A, Meirowitz N. Care bundles for management of obstetrical hemorrhage. *Semin Perinatol*. 2016; 40:99-108.
8. Lagrew D, Lyndon A, Main E, Shields L, Melsop K, Bingham D. *Obstetric hemorrhage toolkit: Improving health care response to obstetric hemorrhage*. (California Maternal Quality Care Collaborative Toolkit to Transform Maternity Care). Stanford, CA: California Maternal Quality Care Collaborative; 2010 Jun.
9. Flo K, Wilsgaard T, Vårtun A, Acharya G. A longitudinal study of the relationship between maternal cardiac output measured by impedance cardiography and uterine artery blood flow in the second half of pregnancy. *BJOG*. 2010; 117:837-844.
10. Begley CM, Gyte GM, Devane D, McGuire W, Weeks A. Active versus expectant management for women in the third stage of labour. *Cochrane Database Syst Rev*. 2015 Mar; 2(3):CD007412.
11. Pacheco LD, Saade GR, Costantine MM, Clark SL, Hankins GD et al. An update on the use of massive transfusion protocols in obstetrics. *Am J Obstet Gynecol*. 2016; 214:340-344.
12. Sarno A, Makhoul J, Smulian JC. Maternal transport in critical care obstetrics. In: Belfort MA, Dildy GA, Saade GR, Phelan JP, Hankins GD, Clark SL, editors. *Critical care obstetrics*. 6th ed. Hoboken, NJ: Blackwell Science; 2017.
13. Stafford I, Dildy G, Clark S, Belfort M. Visually estimated and calculated blood loss in vaginal and cesarean delivery. *Am J Obstet Gynecol*. 2008; 199:519.e1-7.
14. Quantification of blood loss: AWHONN practice brief number 1. *J Obstet Gynecol Neonatal Nurs*. 2015; 44:158-160.
15. O'Leary JL, O'Leary JA. Uterine artery ligation for control of postcesarean section hemorrhage. *ObGyn*. 1974; 43(6):849-853.
16. B-Lynch C, Coker A, Lawal AH, Abu J, Cowen MJ. The B-Lynch surgical technique for the control of massive postpartum haemorrhage: An alternative to hysterectomy? Five cases reported. *Br J Obstet Gynaecol*. 1997; 104:372-375.
17. Matsubara S, Yano H, Ohkuchi A, Kuwata T, Usui R, Suzuki M. Uterine compression sutures for postpartum hemorrhage: An overview. *Acta Obstet Gynecol Scand*. 2013; 92:378-385.
18. Huntington JL, Irving FC, Kellogg FS. Abdominal reposition in acute inversion of the puerperal uterus. *Am J Obstet Gynecol*. 1928; 15:34-40.
19. Haultain FW. The treatment of chronic uterine inversion by abdominal hysterotomy, with a successful case. *Br Med J*. 1901; 2:974-976.
20. Silver RM, Major H. Maternal coagulation disorders and postpartum hemorrhage. *Clin Obstet Gynecol*. 2010; 53:252-264.
21. Woman Trial Collaborators. Effect of early tranexamic acid administration on mortality, hysterectomy, and other morbidities in women with post-partum haemorrhage (WOMAN): An international, randomised, double-blind, placebo-controlled trial. *Lancet*. 2017; 389:2105-2116.
22. Ducloy-Bouthors AS, Jude B, Duhamel A, Broisin F, Huissoud C, Keita-Meyer H et al. High-dose tranexamic acid reduces blood loss in postpartum hemorrhage. *Crit Care*. 2011; 15: R117.
23. Goucher H, Wong CA, Patel SK, Toledo P. Cell salvage in obstetrics [Review]. *Anesth Analg*. 2015; 121:465-468.

# 15

## Acute Abdomen in Pregnancy

**K. Ashley Brandt, DO**

### CONTENTS

## Maternal Physiology

Pregnancy causes significant changes throughout all systems; however, some of the more significant changes are observed in the cardiovascular, hematologic, and respiratory systems. One of the most profound changes that occur is the increase in cardiac output of 30–50% higher than prepregnancy values. An increase in heart rate by up to 15–20 beats per minute must also be considered when interpreting tachycardia in the pregnant patient as this can represent a normal change versus an underlying pathological response.

Plasma volume increases throughout pregnancy until approximately the 34th week of gestation when it plateaus. A physiological anemia is also observed as the small increase in red blood cell volume increases, resulting in a decreased hematocrit level. In the third trimester, a hematocrit level of 31–35% is considered normal. As a result, pregnant patients can lose up to 1200–1500 mL of blood volume before exhibiting the signs and symptoms of hypovolemia (1).

Of the respiratory changes that occur during pregnancy, progesterone stimulates respiratory drive and leads to an increase in tidal volume and minute ventilation. Conversely, the increasing size of the gravid uterus throughout pregnancy leads to a decrease in functional residual capacity and total lung capacity, particular in the third trimester. As a result, pregnancy is associated with a state of relative hyperventilation and mild respiratory alkalosis (2).

A mild leukocytosis is also seen as the white blood cell count increases during pregnancy. Values can range around 12,000/mm³ during pregnancy and can increase to 25,000/mm³ during labor. Other laboratory values such as D-dimer, serum creatinine, and alkaline phosphatase are significantly altered, reducing their reliability in diagnosis in the pregnant patient (2).

The physical examination of the pregnant patient poses an additional challenge due to the changing size of the gravid uterus. During the first trimester until the 12th week of gestation, the uterus is predominantly contained within the bony pelvis. During the second trimester, the enlarged uterus begins to displace other anatomic structures. For example, the appendix is displaced into the right upper abdomen and does not return to its original position until 1–2 weeks postpartum (3).

## Diagnostic Imaging

One of the main concerns regarding the evaluation of a patient presenting with an acute abdomen is the safety of diagnostic imaging tests. It is important to weigh the potential risks of the diagnostic test against any significant harm that may befall the patient if a diagnosis is delayed. Ultrasound is the primary imaging study of choice when initially evaluating a pregnant patient who presents with abdominal pain, as it is readily available, relatively inexpensive, and lacks ionizing radiation. To date, there have been no adverse fetal affects demonstrated with the use of ultrasonography in pregnancy. If ultrasonographic findings are inconclusive, magnetic resonance imaging (MRI) is the next imaging modality of choice. Some advantages of MRI are multiplanar imaging capabilities and the ability to detect and distinguish blood from other fluid collections (4).

The fetal central nervous system is most susceptible during weeks 8–15 as this is a period of rapid neuronal development (2). Radiation doses ranging from 60 to 310 mGy or 6–31 rad (1 mGy = 0.1 rad) may lead to microcephaly, intrauterine growth restriction, and severe mental retardation. After 25 weeks, these risks substantially decrease (5,6). While teratogenic effects are often a concern, ionizing radiation increases the risk of childhood leukemia and other cancers, potentially up to 0.06% with each centigray of exposure (7). Exposure to less than 50 mGy (5 rad) has not been associated with an increase in fetal anomalies or pregnancy loss (8).

As with any diagnostic test or intervention, adequate patient counseling should be performed as to alleviate any concerns the pregnant patient may have regarding harmful effects to the fetus.

## Nonobstetric Causes

### Renal

Renal colic and pyelonephritis is the most common nonobstetric cause for abdominal pain during pregnancy (4). The incidence of pyelonephritis is 1–2% and is the most common nonobstetric cause for hospitalization during pregnancy (9). Pyelonephritis is associated with complications such as preterm labor, recurrent abortions, intrauterine growth restriction, and even fetal death. The treatment for pyelonephritis includes the administration of intravenous antibiotics, generally a broad-spectrum cephalosporin, in addition to providing supportive therapy through intravenous hydration and pain control until clinical improvement is observed. Antibiotic therapy can then be tailored to the specific organism after urine culture sensitivities are obtained. Intravenous antibiotic therapy should be continued for 24–48 hours after the patient becomes afebrile and clinical improvement is seen (for example, the absence of costovertebral tenderness). Treatment with oral antibiotics is recommended for 10–14 days with follow-up urine cultures in each trimester. Recurrent episodes are treated with suppressive therapy for the duration of the pregnancy, typically using 100 mg nitrofurantoin twice daily. If urolithiasis is suspected, a renal ultrasound is warranted. Most renal stones resolve spontaneously, typically as a result of the physiological hydroureter of pregnancy (10). For refractory cases, urological consultation is appropriate for the evaluation of stent placement or nephrostomy tubes. Lithotripsy is contraindicated in pregnancy.

### Appendicitis

Acute appendicitis occurs in 1 in 1500 pregnancies and is the most common nonobstetric surgical emergency (4). Although the incidence of this disease is not increased during pregnancy, the rupture of the appendix occurs up to two to three times more often during pregnancy secondary to delays in diagnosis (11). Classic findings observed in the nonobstetric patient, such as nausea, vomiting, and leukocytosis, are often normal findings in pregnancy. However, despite the altered location of the appendix in

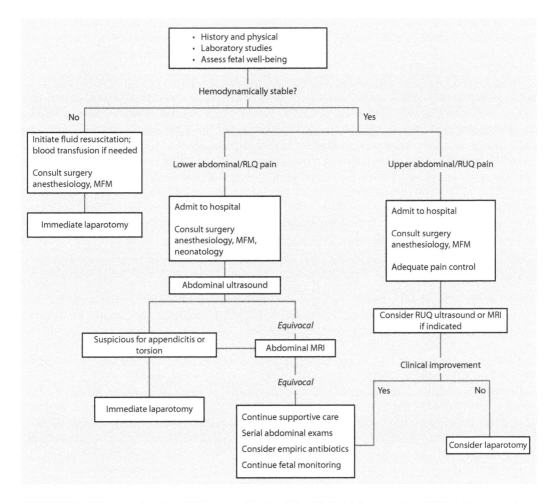

**FIGURE 15.1** Diagnostic algorithm. MFM; maternal fetal medicine; RLQ; right lower quadrant; RUQ; right upper quadrant.

pregnancy, the most reliable symptom is still right lower quadrant pain (2). Ultrasound is the first radio-logical test used with a sensitivity and a specificity value ranging from 50% to 100% and from 33% to 92%, respectively (4). If ultrasonographic findings are equivocal and clinical suspicion is still high, MRI can be used as an additional imaging tool. MRI not only can demonstrate a normal appendix, but can also demonstrate periappendiceal fluid and inflammation (12). The sensitivity and specificity of MRI in the diagnosis of acute appendicitis are 100% and 93%, respectively (13).

Immediate surgical intervention is warranted once the diagnosis of appendicitis is made (Figure 15.1). Over the past two decades, laparoscopy has been increasingly utilized during pregnancy and its safety is adequately demonstrated.

## Acute Cholecystitis

The incidence of gallbladder disease in pregnancy ranges from approximately 1 in 1600 to 1 in 10,000 and is the second most common surgical disorder in pregnancy (11). Over 90% of patients presenting with cholecystitis are affected by gallstones. Well-established risk factors for gallstones include age, female sex, fertility, and obesity. Patients will often present with nausea, vomiting, dyspepsia, intoler-ance to fatty foods, and decreased appetite. Attacks originating in the biliary tract can produce episodic pain that is acute in onset and often triggered by meals. Pain may be localized in the right upper quad-rant, epigastric region and radiate to the shoulder or scapula. Patients will classically present with fever, right upper quadrant pain, and Murphy's sign (tenderness under the liver with deep inspiration). Other disorders to consider in the differential diagnosis is an associated pancreatitis, severe preeclampsia, HELLP syndrome (hemolysis, elevated liver enzymes, and low platelet count), acute fatty liver of pregnancy, and acute hepatitis.

The diagnostic accuracy of a right upper quadrant ultrasound for diagnosing gallstones is 95%, making it the test of choice. Ultrasound findings of acute cholecystitis include gallbladder distension (>5 cm in diameter), wall thickening (>3 mm), pericholcystitc fluid, and wall hyperemia (4). Elevated white blood cell counts and elevated transanimases are often observed. Mildly increased alkaline phosphatase and bilirubin levels are seen in early cholcystitis and bile duct obstruction.

The initial management of acute cholesystitis is nonoperative and supportive therapy, which includes intravenous hydration, pain control, and correction of abnormal laboratory values. If no improvement is seen within 12–24 hours, intravenous antibiotics are warranted. Surgical intervention is often reserved for patients with recurrent episodes of biliary colic, recurrent cholecystitis, choledocholithiasis, and gallstone pancreatitis. Alternatively, endoscopic retrograde cholangiopancreatography is a safe and effective tool in patients with common bile duct stones.

## Acute Pancreatitis

The incidence of pancreatitis during pregnancy is 1 in 1000 to 1 in 10,000 and occurs most often during the third trimester and immediate postpartum period (4,11). Similar to cholecystitis, women with pancreatitis will present with nausea, vomiting, decreased appetite, and epigastric pain radiating to the back. Physical examination is rarely diagnostic, although patients may experience a low-grade fever, tachycardia, and orthostatic hypotension (11). Classic signs such as periumbilical ecchymosis (Cullen's sign) and flank ecchymosis (Turner's sign) are seen with hemorrhagic pancreatitis.

Diagnosis is made by elevations in amylase and lipase levels, although in pregnancy, these levels may normally rise by twofold due to normal physiological changes. Lipase is more specific for the diagnosis as elevated amylase levels can be observed in cholecystitis, bowel obstruction, perforated duodenal ulcer, and liver trauma. Ultrasound can be used to evaluate for the presence of gallstones, abscess, or pancreatic pseudocysts.

The treatment of acute pancreatitis is the same as the treatment for nonpregnant patients, with bowel rest, intravenous hydration, electrolyte repletion, and pain control.

---

## Obstetric Causes

### Placental Abruption

Placental abruption refers to the premature separation of the placenta from the uterine wall prior to the delivery of the fetus. This obstetric emergency complicates approximately 1% of pregnancies (14). Clinical findings are vaginal bleeding associated with abdominal pain, contractions, and uterine tenderness. Fetal indicators of worsening placental abruption often include a nonreassuring fetal heart tracing or persistent fetal bradycardia and even fetal death.

Risk factors that can contribute to placental abruption include increasing parity, advanced maternal age, cigarette smoking, cocaine use, trauma, maternal hypertensive disorders, preterm premature rupture of membranes, multifetal gestation, thrombophilias, uterine malformations, and prior abruption.

The diagnosis of placental abruption is clinical, supported by radiological, laboratory, and pathological studies (14). Ultrasound is less reliable in the diagnosis of placental abruption, as the false-negative rate is high (14). Similarly, changes in laboratory studies, such hypofibrinogenemia, are often not observed in milder cases of abruption and evidence of disseminated intravascular coagulation often suggests severe abruption.

The management of abruption depends on the severity, gestational age, and maternal–fetal status. Once the diagnosis is made, the patient should have intravenous access with a large bore needle, appropriate laboratory studies (complete blood count, type and screen, coagulation studies, fibrinogen), continuous fetal heart monitoring, and tocodynamometry, in addition to notification of both the anesthesia and neonatal teams. Women presenting at or near term should undergo delivery, and the mode of delivery should depend on fetal status and presentation, as well as maternal status.

## Uterine Rupture

Uterine rupture is defined as the complete disruption of all uterine layers (endometrium, myometrium, and serosa) in a nonsurgical setting. The severity of maternal and fetal morbidity depends on the degree of the rupture. The overall incidence of uterine rupture is 1 in 2000 deliveries; it is more common in women who have had previous surgery on the uterus (prior cesarean section or a myomectomy). The location of the prior uterine scar correlates to the incidence of the rupture. For example, in women with one prior cesarean delivery, the overall incidence ranges between 0.5% and 2%; however, in women with a classical or T-shaped incision, the incidence increases up to 4–9% (14).

In women with one prior cesarean section, additional risk factors include multiple prior cesarean deliveries, use of prostaglandin agents for induction of labor, thin uterine scar on ultrasound, fetal macrosomia, single-layer hysterotomy closure, short interpregnancy interval, no prior vaginal delivery, congenital uterine malformations, advanced maternal age, invasive placentation, induced or augmented labor, and postcesarean wound infection (15,16).

Clinical manifestations are observed in both the mother and the fetus. Signs are variable but may include sudden onset vaginal bleeding, persistent abdominal pain, uterine tenderness, loss of fetal station, hematuria, cessation of contractions, and signs of hemodynamic instability. Signs of fetal distress include fetal bradycardia with or without preceding variable or late decelerations. Fetal distress is the most common sign of symptomatic uterine rupture occurring in 33–70% of cases (17).

If the aforementioned signs are observed, a high clinical index of suspicion is warranted, followed by prompt treatment via laparotomy, which will confirm the diagnosis. Surgical findings will reflect the severity of the rupture and range from massive maternal hemorrhage and the expulsion of the fetus into the maternal abdomen or reveal a small disruption in the uterine wall with mild bleeding. The extent of the disruption must be carefully evaluated and assessed for repair. If feasible, it is appropriate to repair the uterus in a multilayered fashion. However, if the uterine defects are significant or massive hemorrhage is occurring with resulting maternal hemodynamic instability, hysterectomy is warranted.

While maternal and/or neonatal mortality are uncommon in cases of uterine rupture, the possibility for significant morbidity is high. Increased rates of genitourinary injury, transfusion, and hysterectomy are higher compared to women who do not experience uterine rupture during a trial of labor after cesarean section. As far as perinatal outcomes are concerned, there is an increase in low 5-minute Apgar scores (<5), decreased umbilical artery pH (<7.0), admission to the neonatal intensive care unit, and hypoxic–ischemic encephalopathy (14).

## Ovarian Torsion

Most adnexal masses encountered in pregnancy are benign and resolve spontaneously (18). Surgery is recommended if the mass is suggestive of malignancy, ovarian torsion is suspected, or patients are clinically symptomatic.

Ovarian torsion in pregnancy is rare, complicating only 7% of pregnancies, with the majority occurring in the first trimester (4). Recognition and surgical intervention is crucial in the early stages of ovarian torsion as delayed diagnosis and treatment may result in ovarian necrosis, sepsis, and possibly preterm labor. The decision to resect as opposed to detorsing the affected ovary is made at the time of confirmatory surgery. If extensive necrosis is identified or there is no discrete ovarian cyst of mass that can be successfully and safely resected, oophorectomy is recommended.

The decision to proceed with laparotomy versus laparoscopy should be individualized and based on the same approach as a nonpregnant patient. As previously stated, laparoscopy has been shown to be a safe and effective method of surgery in pregnancy and would be an appropriate approach in most patients experiencing ovarian torsion.

# REFERENCES

1. American College of Surgeons Committee on Trauma. Trauma in pregnancy and intimate partner violence. In: *Advanced trauma life Support.* 9th ed. Chicago, IL: American College of Surgeons; 2012, pp. 286-297.
2. Schwartz N, Adamczak J, Ludmir J. Surgery during pregnancy. In: Gabbe SG, Niebyl JR, Simpson JL et al., editors. *Obstetrics: Normal and problem pregnancies,* 6th ed. Amsterdam: Elsevier; 2012, pp. 567-580.
3. Wagner JM, McKinney WP, Carpenter JL. Does this patient have appendicitis? *JAMA.* 1996; 276:1589-1594.
4. Masselli G, Derme M, Laghi F, Framarino-dei-Malatesta M, Gualdi G. Evaluating the acute abdomen in the pregnant patient. *Radiol Clin N Am.* 2015; 53:1309-1325.
5. Brent RL. Saving lives and changing family histories: Appropriate counseling of pregnant women and men and women of reproductive age, concerning the risk of diagnostic radiation exposures during and before pregnancy. *Am J Obstet Gynecol.* 2009; 200:4-24.
6. Patel SJ, Reede DL, Katz DS, Subramaniam R, Amorosa JK. Imaging the pregnant patient for nonobstetric conditions: Algorithms and radiation dose considerations. *Radiographics.* 2007; 27:1705-1722.
7. Lee CI, Haims AH, Monico EP, Brink JA, Forman HP. Diagnostic CT scans: Assessment of the patient, physician and radiologist awareness of radiation dose and possible risks. *Radiology.* 2004; 231:393-398.
8. Guidelines for diagnostic imaging during pregnancy and lactation. Committee Opinion No. 723. American College of Obstetricians and Gynecologists. *Obstet Gynecol* 2017; 130:210-216.
9. Plattner MS. Pyelonephritis in pregnancy. *J Perinatol Neonat Nurs.* 1994; 8:20-27.
10. Butler EL, Cox SM, Eberts EG, Cunningham FG. Symptomatic nephrolithiasis complicating pregnancy. *Obstet Gynecol.* 2000; 96:753-756.
11. Speichinger E, Holschneider CH. Chapter 25. Surgical disorders in pregnancy. In: DeCherney AH, Nathan L, Laufer N, Roman AS, editors. *Current diagnosis & treatment: Obstetrics & gynecology,* 11th ed. New York, NY: McGraw-Hill; 2013.
12. Dewhurst C, Beddy P, Pedrosa I. MRI evaluation of acute appendicitis in pregnancy. *J Magn Reson Imaging.* 2013; 37:566-575.
13. Pedrosa I, Lafornara M, Pandharipande PV, Goldsmith JD, Rofsky NM. Pregnant patients suspected of having acute appendicitis: Effect of MR imaging on negative laparotomy rate and appendiceal perforation rate. *Radiology.* 2009; 250:749-757.
14. Francois KE, Foley MR. Antepartum and postpartum hemorrhage. In: Gabbe SG, Niebyl JR, Galan H, Jauniaux E, Landon M, Simpson JL et al., editors. *Obstetrics: Normal and problem pregnancies.,* 6th ed. Amsterdam: Elsevier; 2012, pp. 415-444.
15. Mercer BM, Gilbert S, Landon MB, Spong CY, Leveno KJ, Rouse DJ et al. Labor outcomes with increasing number of prior vaginal births after cesarean delivery. *Obstet Gynecol.* 2008; 111:285-291.
16. Walsh CA, Baxi LV. Rupture of the primagravid uterus: A review of the literature. *Obstet Gynecol Surv.* 2007; 62:327-334.
17. Zwart JJ, Richters JM, Öry F, de Vries JIP, Bloemenkamp KWM, van Roosmalen J. Uterine rupture in the Netherlands: A nationwide population-based cohort study. *BJOG.* 2009; 116:1069-1080.
18. Schwartz N, Timor-Tritsch IE, Wang E. Adenxal masses in pregnancy. *Clin Obstet Gynecol.* 2009; 52:570-585.

# 16

## Trauma

**Hugh M. Ehrenberg, MD**

### CONTENTS

## Introduction

Traumatic injury complicates 6–7% of all pregnancies in the United States (1). Maternal trauma occurs at all gestational ages and is estimated to impact between 350,000 and 500,000 women yearly (2), or approximately 1 in 12 pregnancies (3). The impact of trauma in pregnancy crosses the lines of maternal age, race, and socioeconomic status, with the potential to alter the life of the mother and offspring. Taken together, blunt and penetrating trauma account for approximately 46% (3) of maternal death, making it the leading nonobstetric cause of death. The disease burden without accounting for death remains significant, with a hospitalization rate of 4.1 per 1000 deliveries admitted for injury during pregnancy. Trauma also significantly contributes to fetal and neonatal morbidity and mortality (4–6). Literature-based tabulations of frequencies widely vary due to differences in ascertainment (4–7), but motor vehicle accidents account for approximately 46–70% of trauma in pregnancy (8,9) and now are the leading cause of maternal death in developed countries (10) followed by assault, gunshot wounds, and burns (Table 16.1).

Unfortunately, pregnancy is not protective from exposure to traumatic injury and may itself represent a risk factor for trauma secondary to intimate partner violence (IPV). It is critical to recognize that IPV is an important contributor to many of the mechanisms for injury mentioned. In many studies, IPV represents the second most common etiology of maternal injury (11) and should be screened for with careful attention and taken seriously and have appropriate interventions employed without delay. Risk factors recognized to be associated with IPV include close interval pregnancy and limited education. IPV is not limited to any one socioeconomic group (7).

The obstetric provider must be informed with regard to the potential complications and management pitfalls posed by trauma during pregnancy and be prepared to work with emergency medicine and trauma team members to alter or augment clinical plans for the benefit of the mother and the child. Like many conditions encountered in medicine among nongravid patients, trauma presents a particular set of considerations and complications when the patient is pregnant. The pregnant trauma patient is at increased risk for preterm birth, placental abruption, uterine rupture, preterm premature rupture of the fetal membranes (PPROM), uterine rupture, or fetal demise. Pregnancy will also predictably alter maternal physiology in ways that make the assessment and treatment of a trauma patient more complicated. This chapter will review the epidemiology, pathophysiology, mechanisms, and management considerations of traumatic injury during pregnancy.

TABLE 16.1

Maternal Traumatic Injury and Death

| Injury |  |
|---|---|
| Motor vehicle collision |  |
| Violence and assault | • Gunshots |
|  | • Stabbing |
|  | • Strangulation |
| Falls |  |
| Suicide |  |
| Toxic exposure | • Drug overdose |
|  | • Poisoning |
| Burns |  |
| Drowning |  |

## Patient Assessment

The primary assessment of pregnant trauma patients will follow the Advanced Trauma Life Support principles, with very little alteration in method from the nongravid state (12). The management of maternal trauma requires attention be paid to both mother and fetus as patients, accounting for physiological and anatomical alterations of pregnancy, resulting in a more nuanced approach once the possibility of life-threatening injuries have been evaluated. When considering the effect of a disease state on a pregnant patient, it is sometimes helpful to assess the impact of pregnancy on the disease and the impact of the disease on the pregnancy. This is no less true with trauma. The fetus and mother will each complicate the care of the other, while simultaneously informing providers on the status of each other. It is critical to remember that the gravid patient undergoes physiological changes, many of which begin early in gestation that will affect the outcomes, evaluation, and treatment of maternal trauma. These include increases in resting pulse, pulse pressure, and cardiac stroke volume; quickened respiratory rates and decreased tidal volume; expanded plasma volume; physiological anemia; and a compensated respiratory alkalosis among others (Tables 16.2 and 16.3). It is clear that many of these physiological responses to pregnancy mimic those of a trauma patient. The gravid trauma patient may appear well compensated at presentation, but have a limited physiological reserve with which to cope with her injuries. The resultant underestimation of injury severity, blood loss, or degree of maternal decompensation may delay adequate resuscitative efforts for the mother. Mindfulness of normal hemodynamic changes in pregnancy will aid in acting on appropriate changes outside these parameters for fluid and blood product replacement as well as suspicion for occult injury. At the same time, because many parameters, such as blood pressure, are reduced in normal pregnancy, caregivers must be aware of the lack of plasticity in response to trauma and blood loss and to the limited reserve available to compensate for such loss that the gravid patient may have remaining. The gravid trauma victim may appear relatively stable until the point when she is quite unstable and significantly decompensates rapidly.

TABLE 16.2

Changes in Maternal Physiology in Pregnancy

| Physiological Variable | Change in Pregnancy | Result |
|---|---|---|
| Plasma volume | Increases by 45–50% | Delayed maternal response to minimal blood loss |
| Red cell mass | Increases by 30% | Dilutional anemia |
| Cardiac output | Increases by 30–50% | Delayed maternal response to moderate blood loss |
| Uteroplacental blood flow | 20–30% shunt | Uterine injury may predispose to increased blood loss |
| Uterine mass | Increased | Movement of abdominal contents, supine hypotension |
| Minute ventilation | Increased by 25–30% | Lower $P_aCO_2$, lower buffering capacity |
| Functional residual capacity | Decreased | Predisposes to atelectasis, hypoxemia |
| Gastric emptying | Delayed | Predisposition to aspiration |

TABLE 16.3

Hemodynamic Changes in Pregnancy by Trimester

| Parameter | Nongravid | First Trimester | Second Trimester | Third Trimester |
|---|---|---|---|---|
| Heart rate (beats/min) | 70 | 78 | 82 | 85 |
| Systolic blood pressure (BP) (mm g) | 115 | 112 | 112 | 114 |
| Diastolic BP (mmHg) | 70 | 60 | 63 | 70 |
| Cardiac output (L/min) | 4.5 | 4.5 | 6 | 6 |
| Central venous pressure (mmHg) | 9 | 7.5 | 4 | 3.8 |
| Blood volume (mL) | 4000 | 4200 | 5000 | 5600 |
| Hematocrit (%) | 40 | 36 | 34 | 36 |

The most obvious maternal physiological alteration in pregnancy is the presence of the gravid uterus, which, later in pregnancy, can significantly modify the position of internal organs, exposing them to risk of injury and putting them where the surgeon may not expect. Increases in plasma volume result in more pronounced vascularity within and around the spleen and liver, with increased stroke volume passing through the kidneys. Injuries to these organs may therefore become more grave in minor traumas, making a complete and detailed evaluation important even in seemingly benign circumstances. Lastly, the gravid uterus itself is at significant risk of injury. Early in pregnancy, the fetus and uterus are largely confined to the bony pelvis and as such are protected from much of the risk from both blunt and penetrating trauma. Beyond 12 weeks of gestation, as it grows beyond the confines of the bony pelvis, the uterus is exposed in the abdomen, receiving an increasing proportion of cardiac output with advancing gestation and is at risk for perforation, rupture, and abruption, each of which pose a threat to the life and health of the mother and the fetus. The third-trimester uterine wall is attenuated compared with earlier pregnancy, with higher intrauterine pressures, both of which predispose to the rupture of the organ. Shear forces encountered during sudden deceleration such as are common in motor vehicle collisions represent a root cause for abruptions. These premature separations of placenta occur due to the relative inelasticity of the placental attachment site to the uterus and are second only to maternal death in causing fetal death. Placental abruptions are the most common complication of maternal trauma and a frequent contributor to preterm labor and delivery. The obstetricians' involvement in the clinical assessment and management of a pregnant trauma victim is critical in maintaining the reference points of normal through the lens of pregnancy.

Figure 16.1 suggests an algorithm mapping the coordinated care of the pregnant trauma patient based on injury severity and gestational age, including roles for trauma surgery and obstetrics services. If maternal stability is not readily achieved or if injury severity requires operative management, the participation of the obstetric team will largely depend on gestational age and localization of injuries. Maternal stabilization in these cases is clearly critical for maternal survival and can have a significant influence on fetal well-being as well. Fetal monitoring in the operating room should be delayed until it can be performed without compromising maternal care and stability is established. While the delivery of the viable fetus may be an option for the stable patient, additional surgery for an unstable mother to deliver a fetus in distress will increase maternal morbidity. On the other hand, if cardiovascular compromise cannot be alleviated, there is sometimes a role for the delivery of the fetus at any gestational age as an adjunct to resuscitative efforts. (See Chapters 17 and 18.) Injuries involving the uterus will of course lend themselves to obstetric management, with the aid of trauma surgery.

## Fetus as Patient; Fetal Status as Vital Sign

While the evaluation of the mother is ongoing, the monitoring of the fetal patient may improve outcomes for both mother and offspring. Prior to viable gestational age (23–24 weeks), priority must of course be given to the stabilization of the mother over the monitoring of the fetus. Beyond this point, coordinated efforts to care for the mother while monitoring fetal well-being can aid in the care for both. Firstly, premature delivery related to trauma results in significant contribution to preterm birth. Thirty-six percent

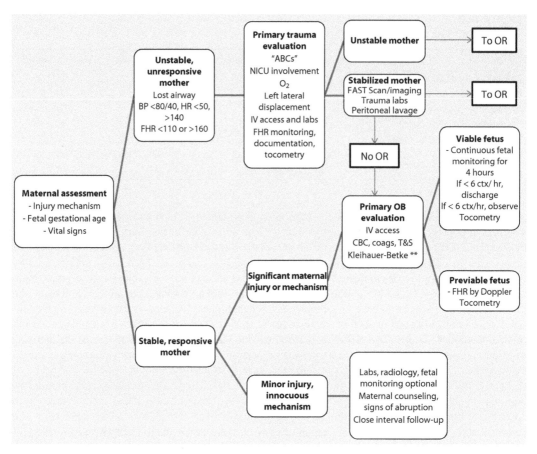

**FIGURE 16.1**  Algorithm: coordinated care of the gravid trauma patient. (Note: ** means or a similar test for fetal–maternal hemorrhage.)

of all pregnant trauma hospital admissions result in delivery during the same hospital stay. Fetal compromise, preterm labor, or early abruptio placentae may occur without significant change in maternal vital signs, and attention paid to mother without any consideration of the fetus may delay intervention as required by these events.

We acknowledge that the monitoring of the fetus may not always be immediately available or feasible, but should be initiated in the viable pregnancy soon after patient arrival and exclusion of life-threatening injury, to allow contemporaneous evaluation with the mother. Patient assessment, in conjunction with trauma specialists or emergency room physicians, of course, includes maternal vital functions. Bedside sonographic assessment, cardiotocography, and obstetric examination, including pelvic evaluation, may not be concomitantly possible with initial maternal trauma evaluation, but should be performed as soon as feasible. Valuable information is obtained via this assessment with regard to fetal number, size and viability status, uterine activity, fundal tenderness, and fetal heart rate patterns. These remain useful adjuncts in assessing for occult bleeding from abruption, preterm labor, PPROM, and fetal well-being, and should be viewed as equally important with second-line maternal evaluations.

Fetal well-being is dependent upon maternal stability, while at the same time, it may be distinctly at risk without maternal change. Literature suggests that the routine assessment of maternal vital signs may not accurately predict fetal status. Variations in maternal status may not correlate with risk for fetal death. It is important to remember that fetal death in utero may be associated with maternal trauma that might otherwise be thought as trivial. Obstetric providers should not assume fetal well-being even with normal maternal vital signs. At the same time, the assessment of fetal well-being may offer insight into the maternal status, as, for example, fetal cardiotocography showing uterine contractions or fetal heart rate decelerations may provide early warning for maternal hypovolemia or decompensation or placental abruption leading to contractions and fetal heart rate changes. In a sense, judiciously assessed during maternal resuscitation, the fetus can act as an in-dwelling invasive cardiac monitor, providing information with regard to central pressures and oxygenation that may not be available through peripheral sources. Taking care to assess both fetal and maternal patients will offer protection to each individual and the mother–baby dyad.

## Selected Maternal and Fetal Diagnostic Studies

Trauma evaluation will inevitably be radiographic. It is important to take fetal exposure into account while performing this evaluation, modifying when possible to limit it, but not to avoid adequate imaging in the name of protecting the fetus from radiation. Estimates of fetal exposures from common radiographic studies are listed in Table 16.4. The use of magnetic resonance imaging is increasing in frequency in trauma centers and is attractive due to the increased level of detail available in imaging with the lack of ionizing radiation. It is notable that despite hesitancy in its use, gadolinium exposure is not known to be harmful to the fetus.

Maternal serum studies such as the Kleihauer–Betke or "fetal dex" should also be sent to assess for fetal–maternal hemorrhage. Debate continues as to the utility in detecting smaller hemorrhage, but large bleeds may prompt additional monitoring of fetal well-being or, in the case of Rh-negative mothers, adjustment in the dose of Rh immunoglobulin (RhoGAM®) to prevent alloimmunization.

Fetal cardiotocographic evaluation (or "nonstress testing" [NST]) is ubiquitous in obstetrics, but serves multiple important purposes in the evaluation of the pregnant trauma patient. NST may reduce the risk of stillbirth from some injuries to pregnant women sustained in blunt trauma that are unique and that pose challenges in their assessment in the injured mother. These include abruption and uterine rupture. Other less dramatic pregnancy outcomes associated with maternal trauma include preterm delivery due to labor or premature rupture of membranes. The duration of risk after injury, or the optimal length of monitoring within that window of risk, remains debatable. The period of greatest risk for adverse pregnancy outcomes, such as labor, abruption, or fetal demise, appears to be the first 24 hours after maternal trauma. In an earlier era, fetal monitoring in trauma cases was somewhat arbitrarily set as 24 hours total, or for 12–24 hours within the first 24 hours after the trauma, but limited utility in risk reduction was demonstrated. Maternal blunt trauma patients have been monitored in the hospital for as long as 24 hours, even without continued suspicion of fetal jeopardy, in an effort to detect women at risk for abruption or stillbirth. In these circumstances, many women are admitted after trauma to acute care locations, such as labor and delivery, and in many centers kept NPO (with an empty stomach with no intake by mouth) and at bed rest during this stay. This represents a patient dissatisfier, and may expose patients to risk of prolonged bed rest (such as venous thromboembolism) for very little gain. More recent literature shows that shorter intervals of monitoring are acceptable for the assessment of obstetric risk after trauma (13). As few as 4 hours of reassuring fetal monitoring may be helpful in reducing the risk of untoward pregnancy outcomes in the settings of minor maternal trauma (5,14).

Laboratory evaluation may also be helpful in stratifying maternal trauma patients into high- and low-risk groups. Complete blood counts, coagulation studies, fibrinogen levels, Kleihauer–Betke or fetal dex

TABLE 16.4

Fetal Radiation Exposures

| Diagnostic Study | Fetal Radiation Exposure |
| --- | --- |
| Chest X-ray | 0.02–0.007 mrad |
| Pelvic X-ray | 100 mrad |
| Head computed tomography (CT) scan | <1 rad |
| Chest CT | <1 rad |
| Abdominal/lumbar spine CT | 3.5 rad |
| Cervical spine CT | <1 rad |
| Pelvic CT | 250 mrad |

evaluation for fetal maternal hemorrhage (15,16), and fibrin split products have all been used to evaluate these patients for evidence of subclinical bleeding in utero leading to coagulopathy. The specificity of fibrin split products or d-dimer levels in the detection of maternal coagulopathy after trauma is extremely low. The utility of these tests is negligible, and they should be avoided. Conversely, care should be taken when evaluating maternal fibrinogen levels. Fibrinogen levels significantly rise in pregnancy (400–650 mg/dL) and levels consistent with nonpregnant normal values (145–400 mg/dL) will represent significant loss of this important protein due to bleeding and the activation of the coagulation cascade. The detection of maternal fetal hemorrhage by laboratory evidence remains of questionable utility as well; subclinical hemorrhage is not typically morbid, and alterations in management have not been shown to improve maternal or fetal outcomes in the setting of mild bleeds (14,17).

## Penetrating Trauma

While the majority of maternal trauma exposure is blunt, special mention should be given to penetrating trauma and pertinent considerations in pregnancy. In one large series, penetrating trauma accounted for just under 10% of trauma admissions. The majority of these were gunshots, followed by stab wounds. Gunshot wounds to the uterus resulted in injury to the fetus in 60–70% of cases and fetal death in 40–65%. When compared to the blunt trauma group, penetrating trauma was extremely uncommon, but associated with a markedly increased risk for maternal morbidity, longer length of stay, and maternal and fetal mortality (12). Fetal death risk may be as high as 71% with gunshot injuries and 42% with stab wounds (10) (Table 16.5).

The most common maternal complication from penetrating trauma was ileus (57%), although bowel injury with penetrating trauma becomes less common as pregnancy progresses due to the space-occupying nature of the gravid uterus. Conversely, upper abdominal stab wounds may result in more complicated bowel injuries due to the upward displacement of the small bowel in its entirety at that time. The risk of direct uterine injury is largely limited to the second and third trimesters, as the first trimester uterus is a pelvic organ, protected from such injury by the bony pelvis. The risk of fetal death due to uterine stab wounds remains low in the later two trimesters due to the development of uterine musculature capable of absorbing most of wounding energy in these cases, and there is limited protection afforded to other abdominal organs by the presence of the expanded gravid uterus (1,10). Unfortunately, the same cannot be said for gunshot wounds. The variable trajectory taken by the projectile after abdominal penetration subjects all organs to risk of injury, particularly with the fragmentation of the ammunition after impact with bone (18,19).

The surgical treatment of penetrating trauma will be employed in many cases, particularly after gunshot wounds. Proceeding with emergent cesarean delivery, or cesarean hysterectomy may be warranted both for the preservation of the viable infant and maternal well-being independently from any surgical exploration. Indications for cesarean include maternal shock, threat to life from exsanguination, uterine injury that cannot be repaired, pregnancy near term, maternal death, and nonreassuring fetal status.

## Prevention

Physicians are not powerless to mitigate the effects of maternal trauma on the well-being of mother and child. While it may be beyond the scope of this volume to discuss prevention per se, it is crucial to recognize the power of the physician–patient relationship, and the potential obstetric providers have to identify

TABLE 16.5

Penetrating Trauma and Pregnancy Outcomes

| Outcome | Penetrating Trauma (n = 30) (%) | Blunt Trauma (n = 291) (%) | Adjusted OR (95% CI) | Adjusted p Value |
|---|---|---|---|---|
| Maternal mortality | 7 | 2 | 7.29 (0.6579) | 0.09 |
| Fetal mortality | 73 | 10 | 34 (11–124) | <0.0001 |
| Maternal morbidity | 66 | 10 | 25 (9–79) | <0.0001 |

*Note:* CI, confidence interval; OR, odds ratio.

TABLE 16.6

Seatbelt Use and Pregnancy Outcomes

| Outcome | Unrestrained (*n* = 1349) # (%) | Restrained (*n* = 1243) # (%) | Relative Risk | 95% CI |
|---|---|---|---|---|
| Birth weight < 2500 g | 62 (4.6) | 36 (2.9) | 1.9 | 1.2–2.9 |
| Delivery within 48 hours of MVC | 33 (2.5) | 11 (0.9) | 2.3 | 1.1–4.9 |
| Fetal death | 7 (0.5) | 2 (0.2) | 4.1 | 0.8–20.3 |
| Abruption | 10 (0.7) | 11 (0.9) | 0.9 | 0.4–2.2 |
| Cesarean delivery | 219 (16.2) | 226 (18.2) | 1.0 | 0.8–1.2 |
| Respiratory distress | 7 (0.5) | 9 (0.7) | 0.9 | 0.3–2.7 |

*Note:* #, refers to number of study subjects in each group, as in #/% of the whole; MVC, motor vehicle collision.

and modify behaviors, relationships, and exposures that may increase the likelihood of maternal trauma. Physicians should use prenatal care as an opportunity to counsel with regard to the correct use of seatbelts (Table 16.6). By teaching that the three-point restraint should be worn with the lap belt across the thighs under the abdomen and the shoulder belt between the breasts, physicians may reduce the severity of traumatic injuries. Screening for IPV may provide just the right motivation to safety that the patient is looking for at the right moment, reducing exposure to danger.

## Coordinated Approach

Trauma in pregnancy presents a challenge in management for both the obstetrician and the trauma surgeon. Careful coordination of care, with a team approach toward the mother baby unit and her needs, will aide in improving outcomes for both patients. The time spent in the prevention of traumatic injuries and the assessment of risk for IPV during the course of prenatal care may yield reduced risk for all parties.

## REFERENCES

1. Brown HL. Trauma in pregnancy. *Obstet Gynecol.* 2009; 114(1):147-160.
2. John PR, Shiozawa A, Haut ER, Efron DT, Haider A, Cornwell III EE et al. An assessment of the impact of pregnancy on trauma mortality. *Surgery.* 2011; 149(1):94-98.
3. Hill CC, Pickinpaugh J. Trauma and surgical emergencies in the obstetric patient. *Surg Clin North Am.* 2008; 88(2):421-440, viii.
4. Aniuliene R et al. Trauma in pregnancy: Complications, outcomes, and treatment. *Medicina (Kaunas).* 2006; 42(7):586-591.
5. Pak LL, Reece EA, Chan L. Is adverse pregnancy outcome predictable after blunt abdominal trauma? *Am J Obstet Gynecol.* 1998; 179(5):1140-1144.
6. Wali UJ, Andrews V, Banerjee S. Abdominal trauma in pregnancy. *Injury.* 2012; 43(7):1223.
7. Wyant AR, Collett D. Trauma in pregnancy: Diagnosis and management of two patients in one. *JAAPA.* 2013; 26(5):24-29.
8. Wolf ME, Alexander BH, Rivara FP, Hickok DE, Maier RV, Starzyk PM. A retrospective cohort study of seatbelt use and pregnancy outcome after a motor vehicle crash. *J Trauma.* 1993; 34(1):116-119.
9. Weiss HB, Strotmeyer S. Characteristics of pregnant women in motor vehicle crashes. *Inj Prev.* 2002; 8(3):207-210.
10. Brown S, Mozurkewich E. Trauma during pregnancy. *Obstet Gynecol Clin North Am.* 2013; 40(1):47-57.
11. Mirza FG, Devine PC, Gaddipati S. Trauma in pregnancy: A systematic approach. *Am J Perinatol.* 2010; 27(7):579-586.
12. Petrone P, Talving P, Browdy T, Teixeira PG, Fisher O, Lozornio A et al. Abdominal injuries in pregnancy: A 155-month study at two level 1 trauma centers. *Injury.* 2011; 42(1):47-49.

13. Curet MJ, Schermer CR, Demarest GB, Bieneik EJ, Curet LB, Rozycki GS et al. Predictors of outcome in trauma during pregnancy: Identification of patients who can be monitored for less than 6 hours. *J Trauma.* 2000; 49(1):18-24; discussion 24-25.

14. Towery R, English TP, Wisner D. Evaluation of pregnant women after blunt injury. *J Trauma.* 1993; 35(5):731-735; discussion 735-736.

15. Dhanraj D, Lambers D. The incidences of positive Kleihauer–Betke test in low-risk pregnancies and maternal trauma patients. *Am J Obstet Gynecol.* 2004; 190(5):1461-1463.

16. Muench MV, Baschat AA, Reddy UM, Mighty HE, Weiner CP, Scalea TM et al. Kleihauer–Betke testing is important in all cases of maternal trauma. *J Trauma.* 2004; 57(5):1094-1098.

17. Williams JK, McClain L, Rosemurgy AS, Colorado NM. Evaluation of blunt abdominal trauma in the third trimester of pregnancy: Maternal and fetal considerations. *Obstet Gynecol.* 1990; 75(1):33-37.

18. Goff BA, Muntz HG. Gunshot wounds to the gravid uterus: A case report. *J Reprod Med.* 1990; 35(4):436-438.

19. Carugno JA, Rodriguez A, Brito J, Cabrera C. Gunshot wound to the gravid uterus with non-lethal fetal injury. *J Emerg Med.* 2008; 35(1):43-45.

# 17

## Maternal Resuscitation

Nicole Yonke, MD, MPH and Lawrence Leeman, MD, MPH

CONTENTS

## Introduction

Maternal collapse and cardiopulmonary resuscitation is fortunately rare and many maternity care providers have minimal experience. In one study, only 15% of maternity care providers would have passed Advanced Cardiac Life Support (ACLS), and many are unfamiliar with modifications of ACLS recommended during pregnancy (1). Resuscitation in pregnant women is unique because there are two patients, the pregnant woman and her fetus.

## Identification of Collapse and Cardiopulmonary Arrest

Women with cardiopulmonary arrest may be found anywhere. Since many etiologies of arrest commonly occur during or immediately after labor, including obstetrical hemorrhage, amniotic fluid embolism, sepsis, and anesthesia complications, nurses or other hospital staff may be the first to find her and activate the emergency response system. Other etiologies, including pulmonary embolism, peripartum cardiomyopathy, or myocardial infarction, may occur at home or anywhere in the community. The National Partnership for Maternal Safety recommends that all cases of cardiac arrest and maternal near misses are reviewed at each maternity unit (2). Since maternal collapse is rare, training drills are another essential component of preparing for and preventing maternal collapse. In a study of simulated maternal collapse, over half of teams failed to perform left uterine displacement (LUD), an essential component of effective cardiopulmonary resuscitation (3). Half of the teams also used incorrect ventilation and compression rates (3). Instructions on how to perform training drills at your institution are available from the National Partnership for Maternal Safety and the California Maternal Quality Care Collaborative (4,5). There is no standard criteria for training maternity care providers or who should be trained in advanced cardiac life support. Two maternity care courses that include maternal resuscitation are Advanced Life Support for Obstetrics (ALSO) and Managing Obstetrics Emergencies and Trauma (MOET) (6,7).

## Epidemiology and Etiology of Maternal Collapse

Cardiac arrest occurred in 1 in 12,000 deliveries in the United States between 1998 and 2001 (8,9). Almost 60% of pregnant women suffering from cardiopulmonary collapse survived to hospital discharge, compared to only 22.3% of all hospitalized adults experiencing an arrest (9,10). Postpartum and antepartum hemorrhage are the most common proximate causes of maternal arrest, accounting for 28 and 17% of arrests, respectively (9). Approximately 1 in 1000 women with an obstetrical hemorrhage will have a cardiac arrest (9). Heart failure, amniotic fluid embolus, sepsis, and anesthetic complications are the next most common causes of arrest (9). Other etiologies of collapse are listed in Table 17.1. Women with preexisting cardiac disease, pulmonary hypertension, liver disease, systemic lupus erythematous, and malignancy are at highest risk for cardiac arrest (9). Obstetric conditions increasing the odds of cardiac arrest are cesarean delivery (odds ratio [OR] 6.7; 99% confidence interval [CI] 5.4–8.3), severe preeclampsia (OR 6.5; 99% CI 5.0–8.3), and placenta previa (OR 4.4; 99% CI 2.9–6.5) (9).

Although hemorrhage is the most common cause of collapse, cardiovascular disease is the most common cause of death, followed by preeclampsia or eclampsia, hemorrhage, venous thromboembolism, and amniotic fluid embolus (11). Mortality is not equally distributed, with race and age as important risk factors. Non-Hispanic black women are 3.2 times more likely to die during pregnancy compared to non-Hispanic white women, having a pregnancy related mortality of 38.9 per 100,000 live births compared to 16.0 per 100,000 for all women (12). Mortality is also higher for women older than 35 years and with Medicaid coverage (9).

## Cardiopulmonary Resuscitation

### Prediction and Preparation for Collapse

One of the key components of preparing for cardiopulmonary resuscitation during pregnancy is identifying women at risk for collapse based on risk factors and using the risk assessment of tools for timely recognition of life-threatening conditions (13). Team members will vary depending on location and resources available. In tertiary care centers, teams may be composed of an intensivist, anesthesiologist, obstetrician, neonatology, nursing, and possibly respiratory therapy. In a rural hospital, it may be essential for an obstetrician or family physician in labor and delivery to perform cardiopulmonary resuscitation (CPR) with anyone else on site including, potentially, an emergency room physician or nurse anesthetist. Practicing with all key team members will be an important component of successful resuscitation (14).

Communication between team members is essential. Closed-loop communication should be used to ensure that directions are understood and followed. Time-outs during resuscitation can be used to

TABLE 17.1

Etiologies of Maternal Arrest

| A | Anesthetic complications, accidents/trauma |
|---|---|
| B | Bleeding—Placental attachment disorders, abruption, uterine rupture |
| C | Cardiovascular—Heart failure, cardiomyopathy, congenital heart disease, aortic dissection/rupture, myocardial infarction |
| D | Drugs—Magnesium toxicity, anaphylaxis, drug errors/overdose |
| E | Embolic causes—Amniotic fluid embolus, venous thromboembolism, pulmonary embolism |
| F | Fever—Sepsis |
| G | General—Hs and Ts |
| H | Hypertension—Preeclampsia/eclampsia, HELLP (hemolysis, elevated liver enzymes, low platelets) |

*Source:* Jeejeebhoy, F. M. et al., *Circulation*, 132, 1747–1773, Table 1, 2015.

summarize events and determine possible diagnosis and interventions (15). Communicating with other key teams such as the neonatal team is also essential. Roles should be assigned to each team member including team leader, timekeeper/documenter, airway, multiple people to rotate chest compressions after 2 minutes, and someone to perform LUD (16).

## Review of Basic Life Support and Advanced Cardiac Life Support

Cardiac arrest in pregnancy is managed following the American Heart Association (AHA) basic life support (BLS) and ACLS algorithms with a few changes related to maternal physiology. Table 17.2 summarizes these recommendations. An unstable patient should be placed in the left lateral decubitus position to relieve aortocaval compression and intravenous (IV) access should be placed above the diaphragm to avoid obstruction from the uterus (13).

The emergency response system activating maternal and neonatal code teams should be initiated at the time of arrest. The time of arrest should be recorded since this helps determine when a perimortem cesarean delivery (PMCD) should be performed. Table 17.3 includes a checklist of key tasks that should be completed in the first minutes of cardiac arrest. The C (Circulation/Compressions), A (airway), B (breathing) algorithm from the AHA should be followed. Please see Figures 17.1 and 17.2 for the cardiac arrest in pregnancy algorithms.

Chest compressions should be performed on a hard surface by deflating air-filled beds or using a backboard on a soft surface if feasible and it does not delay care (13). The hands should be placed in the normal position in the middle of the chest on the lower half of the sternum. It was previously recommend that the hands be placed higher on the sternum during pregnancy; however, magnetic resonance imaging studies have since shown that the heart is not significantly displaced in pregnancy (13,17). The compression depth should be at least 2 in. and performed at a rate of 100 per minute in order to be effective (13). Interruptions to compressions should be limited, and the chest should be allowed to completely recoil. The compression–ventilation ratio is 30:2. One hundred percent oxygen should be administered at ≥15 L/minute with a bag-valve mask or advanced airway with sufficient volume to cause chest rise. Women should be cared for at the scene of collapse rather than being transported to an operating room during arrest since the quality of compressions is usually inadequate during transport (18).

Pregnant women should not be placed in left lateral tilt using a wedge to decrease aortocaval compression during resuscitation, as was previously recommended by the AHA. Instead, pregnant women should be placed supine for chest compressions, like any other adult (13). Tilting pregnant women results in patients sliding off the incline, does not completely decrease aortocaval compression, and, most importantly, results in reduced force in compressions, making them less effective (19). Instead of left lateral tilt, manual LUD should be performed on any women with a uterus palpated at or above the umbilicus or with a known gestational age of ≥20 weeks. If it is unclear where the fundus is located or the gestational age is unknown, LUD should still be attempted (13). LUD makes performing chest compressions easier than tilt and allows easier access to the airway. Although LUD has not been specifically studied in cardiac arrest, it has been shown to decrease hypotension in cesarean deliveries (20). To perform LUD, the uterus should be lifted up and leftward off the maternal vessels (Figure 17.3).

TABLE 17.2

Summary of Resuscitation Recommendations during Pregnancy

- Perform continuous manual LUD to relieve aortocaval compression anytime the uterus is palpated at or above the umbilicus.
- Do not place pregnant women in left tilt during compressions.
- Place the hands in the usual position for chest compressions in the lower half of the sternum.
- Use routine ACLS medications and defibrillation; no pregnancy-specific changes are required.
- Perform PMCD/resuscitative hysterotomy if spontaneous return of circulation does not occur within 4 minutes of arrest.

TABLE 17.3

Checklist of Key Tasks during the First Minutes of In-House Maternal Cardiac Arrest

| | |
|---|---|
| Call for help! | ☐ Call "OB code" |
| | ☐ Call neonatal team |
| Start CPR | ☐ Immediate BLS |
| | ☐ Automated external defibrillator (AED)/defibrillator |
| | ☐ Adult code cart |
| | ☐ Adult airway equipment |
| | ☐ Backboard |
| | ☐ Scalpel/cesarean pack |
| | ☐ Assign timer/documenter |
| C—Circulation | ☐ Manual LUD |
| Chest Compressions | ☐ Hands midsternum |
| | ☐ 100 compressions/minute |
| | ☐ Push Hard! Push Fast! |
| | ☐ Change compressors every 2 minutes |
| | ☐ Obtain IV access above diaphragm |
| A—Airway | ☐ Chin left/jaw thrust |
| | ☐ 100% $O_2$ at 10–15 L/minute |
| | ☐ Use self-inflating bag mask |
| | ☐ Oral |
| | ☐ Experienced personnel: Intubation with 6–7.0 ETT |
| | ☐ Supraglottic airway (LMA) |
| | ☐ Do not interrupt chest compressions! |
| B—Breathing | ☐ If intubated: 10 breaths per minute (500–700 mL per breath) |
| | ☐ If not intubated: 30 compressions to 2 breaths |
| | ☐ Administer each breath over 1 s |
| D—Defibrillate | ☐ Pads front and back |
| | ☐ Use AED or analyze/defibrillate every 2 minutes |
| | ☐ Immediately resume CPR for 2 minutes |
| | ☐ Prepare for delivery |
| E—Extract fetus | ☐ Aim for incision by 4 minutes |
| | ☐ Aim for fetal delivery by 5 minutes |

*Source:* Lipman, S. et al., The Society for Obstetric Anesthesia and Perinatology consensus statement on the management of cardiac arrest in pregnancy, *Anesthesia & Analgesia*, 118, 5, 1003–1016, 2014. With permission.

ACLS medications are used routinely and not withheld due to concerns about their use in pregnancy or teratogenicity. Although physiological changes of pregnancy may affect medication pharmacology, there are no studies evaluating this, and no changes are recommended (13). Amiodarone (300 mg) is recommended for shock-resistant ventricular fibrillation and tachycardia (13). Epinephrine (1 mg IV) should be given every 3–5 minutes during cardiac arrest per ACLS protocol (13). Defibrillation is performed at 120–200 J with the lateral pad underneath the breast tissue for ventricular fibrillation or pulseless ventricular tachycardia (13). Energy should be escalated if it is not effective, as it is in nonpregnant patients.

Possible etiologies of arrest (see Table 17.1) should be immediately addressed to prevent and or possibly reverse cardiac arrest. If magnesium is suspected as a possible cause of arrest, it should be stopped and 1 g of calcium gluconate or calcium chloride should be intravenously given over 2 minutes (21). Lipid emulsion may be administered if cardiac arrest due to local anesthetic is suspected with an initial bolus of 20% lipid emulsion at 1.5 mL/kg of ideal body weight with maintenance infusion of 0.25 mL/kg ideal body weight per minute (15).

The goal of resuscitation is the return of spontaneous circulation (ROSC). Resuscitation should concentrate on the mother; fetal assessment should not be performed during resuscitation as it does not help guide therapy. Monitors can be removed if this does not delay other resuscitative measures (13).

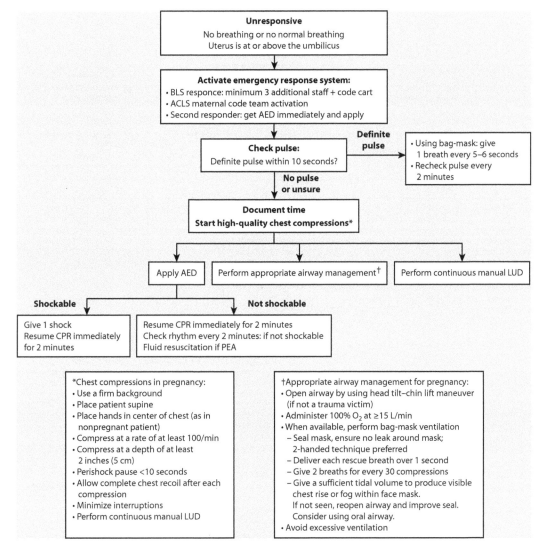

**FIGURE 17.1** Cardiac arrest in pregnancy in-hospital BLS algorithm: simultaneous C-A-B-U (chest compressions/current airway-breathing-uterine displacement). ACLS, advanced cardiovascular life support; AED, automated external defibrillator; CPR, cardiopulmonary resuscitation; LUD, left uterine displacement; PEA, pulseless electric activity. (From Jeejeebhoy, F. M. et al., *Circulation*, 132, 1747–1773, 2015. With permission.)

Fetal monitoring can resume after ROSC. Defibrillation can be performed if fetal monitors are present and should not be delayed. Chest compressions should be immediately resumed after delivery of a shock, without checking for a pulse first. Figure 17.2 reviews the ACLS algorithm.

Hypoxemia develops more rapidly in pregnant patients due to increased metabolic rates and may be a cause of cardiac arrest. Due to airway changes, intubation is more difficult during pregnancy. It is recommended that no more than two attempts at intubation by an experienced provider be made before a supraglottic airway such as a laryngeal mask airway (LMA) is placed in order to avoid the prolonged interruption of chest compressions or airway trauma with multiple attempts. A cricothyroidotomy is the last option for obtaining an airway (13). Cricoid pressure is no longer routinely recommended during the intubation of pregnant patients as it does not prevent aspiration, but may be used at provider discretion (13). If an endotracheal tube is placed, continuous capnography should be used to confirm correct placement and monitor the effectiveness of CPR (13).

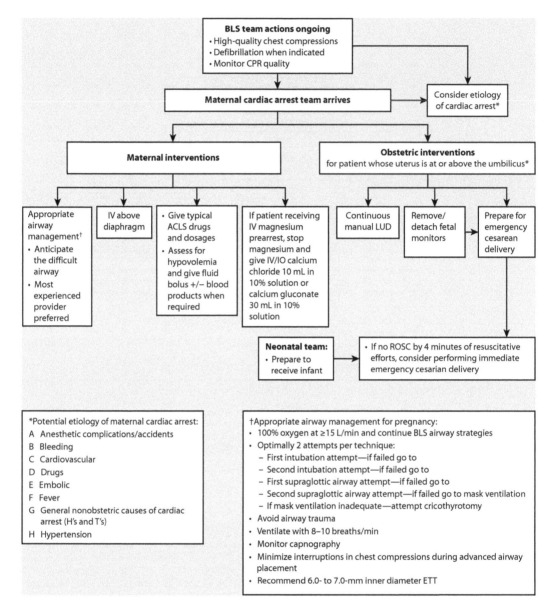

**FIGURE 17.2** Cardiac arrest in pregnancy in-hospital ACLS algorithm. BLS, basic life support; CPR, cardiopulmonary resuscitation; ETT, endotracheal tube; IO, intraosseous; IV, intravenous; LUD, left uterine displacement; ROSC, return of spontaneous circulation. (From Jeejeebhoy, F. M. et al., *Circulation*, 132, 1747–1773, 2015. With permission.)

## Perimortem Cesarean Delivery versus Resuscitative Hysterotomy

The AHA recommends PMCD by 4 minutes if there is no ROSC at a gestational age of ≥20–24 weeks or with a uterus at or above the umbilicus. Aortocaval compression by the uterus decreases cardiac output with compressions to approximately 10%, compared to the normal 30% (16,22). PMCD should be performed at the site of arrest to minimize interruptions in CPR and the delays inherent in transporting to an operating room (13). PMCD increases the likelihood of ROSC in women with a uterine fundus palpable

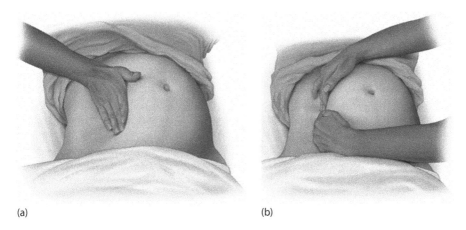

(a)           (b)

FIGURE 17.3 Manual LUD using (a) a one-handed and (b) a two-handed technique. (From Lavonas, E. J. et al., *Circulation*, 132, S501–S518, 2015. With permission.)

at or above the umbilicus by emptying the uterus, relieving aortocaval compression and increasing cardiac output. Operative vaginal delivery with forceps or vacuum is the preferred option for delivery if the cervix is completely dilated and fetal station is low (13).

The 4-minute rule originates from the assumption that normal nonpregnant adults begin to experience anoxic brain injury at 4–6 minutes postarrest (22). However, pregnant women have higher metabolisms and increased oxygen consumption, increasing their risk prior to these 4 minutes (22). Benson et al. (22) argue that there is no evidence to support that 4-minute rule as their review found that survival decreases in a linear fashion, and it did not have a large drop at 4 minutes as suggested by the "4-minute rule" cesarean section. The birth of an infant at 1 minute is also not attainable in studies, making delivery by 5 minutes unrealistic (22). They recommend a change to "deliver the baby as quickly as possible for both maternal and fetal benefit" (22). Both Benson et al. (22) and Rose et al. (23) propose a paradigm shift from PMCD to resuscitative hysterotomy, advocating that hysterotomy be immediately performed in maternal cardiac arrest to enhance the chance of maternal and fetal outcomes. However, this topic remains controversial. Lipman et al. (24) argue that the term *hysterotomy* can be confusing for nonobstetric providers and only means making an incision as opposed to actually emptying the uterus (24). They are also concerned that trying to interpret a cardiac rhythm to determine if immediate PMCD should be performed will be challenging. They recommend following the AHA guidelines with PMCD at 4 minutes. Rose et al. (25) responded that the concern with PMCD is that providers will not view PMCD as a part of resuscitation (25). Whether called resuscitative hysterotomy or PMCD, emptying the uterus to restore circulation is a key component of maternal resuscitation for both maternal and fetal survivals (13).

## Postresuscitative Care

Once the woman is stabilized with a pulse and blood pressure, care should include plans for transfer after the event. Women should be transferred to an intensive care unit either at the facility where the arrest occurred or there should be a plan to transfer to a facility with a higher level of care. If she remains pregnant postarrest and the fetus is above the gestational age of viability, then continuous fetal monitoring should be performed (13). Premature live born neonates or women at risk of pre-term delivery under 34–36 weeks should be transferred to a facility with a neonatal intensive care unit. Therapeutic hypothermia has minimal evidence supporting its use in pregnancy and the decision to use therapeutic hypothermia can be made on a case-by-case basis (13).

## Summary

Most maternity care or emergency medicine providers will rarely encounter maternal cardiac arrest unless they are working at a trauma center, making drills essential to provide practice of incorporating the changes to resuscitation required in pregnancy. Multiple national organizations have guidelines on how to prepare for obstetric emergencies. Etiologies for maternal collapse should be considered as cardiopulmonary resuscitation is initiated and interventions targeted toward reversible causes. BLS and ACLS algorithms including medications and defibrillation should be performed as in a nonpregnant patient, with the addition of LUD. If ROSC does not occur in 4 minutes, a PMCD should be immediately performed to release aortocaval compression and increase cardiac output with chest compressions. Preparing for these emergencies can help decrease maternal morbidity and mortality in the United States.

## REFERENCES

1. Cohen SE, Andes LC, Carvalho B. Assessment of knowledge regarding cardiopulmonary resuscitation of pregnant women. *Int J Obstet Anesth.* 2008; 17(1):20-25.
2. D'Alton ME, Main EK, Menard MK, Levy BS. The National Partnership for Maternal Safety. *Obstet Gynecol.* 2014; 123(5):973-977.
3. Lipman SS, Daniels KI, Carvalho B, Arafeh J, Harney K, Puck A et al. Deficits in the provision of cardiopulmonary resuscitation during simulated obstetric crises. *Am J Obstet Gynecol.* 2010; 203(2):179e1-179e5.
4. California Maternal Quality Care Collaborative. *About us.* Stanford, CA: California Maternal Quality Care Collaborative; 2016. Available from: https://www.cmqcc.org/.
5. Council on Patient Safety in Women's Health Care. *Safe health care for every woman.* Washington, DC: Council on Patient Safety in Women's Health Care; 2015. Available from: http://www.safehealthcarefor everywoman.org/.
6. Advanced Life Support Group. *Managing obstetric emergencies and trauma.* Manchester: Advanced Life Support Group; 2016. Available from: http://www.alsg.org/uk/MOET.
7. American Academy of Family Physicians. *Advanced Life Support in Obstetrics* (ALSO). Leawood, KS: American Academy of Family Physicians; 2016. Available from: http://www.aafp.org/cme/programs/also.html.
8. Neggers YH. Trends in maternal mortality in the United States. *Reprod Toxicol.* 2016; 64:72-76.
9. Mhyre JM, Tsen LC, Einav S, Kuklina EV, Leffert LR, Bateman BT. Cardiac arrest during hospitalization for delivery in the United States, 1998–2011. *Anesthesiology.* 2014; 120(4):810-818.
10. Girotra S, Nallamothu BK, Spertus JA, Li Y, Krumholz HM, Chan PS et al. Trends in survival after in-hospital cardiac arrest. *N Engl J Med.* 2012; 367(20):1912-1920.
11. Main EK, McCain CL, Morton CH, Holtby S, Lawton ES. Pregnancy-related mortality in California: Causes, characteristics, and improvement opportunities. *Obstet Gynecol.* 2015; 125(4):938-947.
12. Creanga AA, Berg CJ, Syverson C, Seed K, Bruce FC, Callaghan WM. Pregnancy-related mortality in the United States, 2006–2010. *Obstet Gynecol.* 2015; 125(1):5-12.
13. Jeejeebhoy FM, Zelop CM, Lipman S, Carvalho B, Joglar J, Mhyre JM et al. Cardiac arrest in pregnancy: A scientific statement from the American Heart Association. *Circulation.* 2015; 132(18):1747-1773.
14. Pandian R, Mathur M, Mathur D. Impact of "fire drill" training and dedicated obstetric resuscitation code in improving fetomaternal outcome following cardiac arrest in a tertiary referral hospital setting in Singapore. *Arch Gynecol Obstet.* 2015; 291(4):945-949.
15. Lipman S, Cohen S, Einav S, Jeejeebhoy F, Mhyre JM, Morrison LJ et al. The Society for Obstetric Anesthesia and Perinatology consensus statement on the management of cardiac arrest in pregnancy. *Anesth Analg.* 2014; 118(5):1003-1016.
16. Lavonas EJ, Drennan IR, Gabrielli A, Heffner AC, Hoyte CO, Orkin AM et al. Part 10: Special circumstances of resuscitation: 2015 American Heart Association guidelines update for cardiopulmonary resuscitation and emergency cardiovascular care. *Circulation.* 2015; 132(18 Suppl 2):S501-S518.
17. Holmes S, Kirkpatrick ID, Zelop CM, Jassal DS. MRI evaluation of maternal cardiac displacement in pregnancy: Implications for cardiopulmonary resuscitation. *Am J Obstet Gynecol.* 2015; 213(3):401e1-401e5.

18. Lipman SS, Wong JY, Arafeh J, Cohen SE, Carvalho B. Transport decreases the quality of cardiopulmonary resuscitation during simulated maternal cardiac arrest. *Anesth Analg.* 2013; 116(1):162-167.

19. Jeejeebhoy F, Windrim R. Management of cardiac arrest in pregnancy. *Best Pract Res Clin Obstet Gynecol.* 2014; 28(4):607-618.

20. Kundra P, Khanna S, Habeebullah S, Ravishankar M. Manual displacement of the uterus during Caesarean section. *Anaesthesia.* 2007; 62(5):460-465.

21. Leeman L, Dresang LT, Fontaine P. Hypertensive disorders of pregnancy. *Am Fam Physician.* 2016; 93(2):121-127.

22. Benson MD, Padovano A, Bourjeily G, Zhou Y. Maternal collapse: Challenging the four-minute rule. *EBioMedicine.* 2016; 6:253-257.

23. Rose CH, Faksh A, Traynor KD, Cabrera D, Arendt KW, Brost BC. Challenging the 4- to 5-minute rule: From perimortem cesarean to resuscitative hysterotomy. *Am J Obstet Gynecol.* 2015; 213(5):653-656.

24. Lipman SS, Cohen S, Mhyre J, Carvalho B, Einav S, Arafeh J et al. Challenging the 4- to 5-minute rule: From perimortem cesarean to resuscitative hysterotomy. *Am J Obstet Gynecol.* 2016; 215(1):129-131.

25. Rose CH, Faksh A, Traynor KD, Cabrera D, Arendt KW, Brost BC. Reply. *Am J Obstet Gynecol.* 2016; 215(1):131.

# 18

## Perimortem Cesarean Delivery

**Stephanie Martin, DO and Nicole Ruddock Hall, MD**

CONTENTS

## Introduction

Cardiopulmonary arrest in pregnancy is a rare emergency which occurs in approximately 1/12,000 admissions for delivery (1). A perimortem cesarean delivery (PMCD) is one which occurs after the initiation of cardiopulmonary resuscitation (CPR). Guidelines for the management of the pregnant patient after cardiac arrest are largely based on expert opinion and case series without the benefit of randomized controlled trials. It is further complicated by the presence of two patients, the mother and fetus, as well as the physiological changes unique to pregnancy. Published reports of PMCD are affected by selection bias, in which favorable outcomes are more likely to be published.

There are specific considerations which influence the approach to resuscitation and may affect maternal and fetal outcomes. These include the etiology of the arrest, the estimated gestational age of the fetus, and whether the arrest occurred pre- or in-hospital. The resuscitation of the pregnant patient requires a multidisciplinary team to treat the mother, deliver the fetus, and resuscitate the neonate if appropriate. Neurological injury of the mother begins about 6 minutes after the cessation of cerebral blood flow (2). Cesarean delivery and uterine evacuation ultimately optimize efforts for maternal resuscitation and should be completed within 5 minutes of cardiac arrest (3).

## Etiology

The most common obstetric causes of cardiopulmonary arrest in pregnancy are hemorrhage (17%), hypertensive disorders of pregnancy (16%), idiopathic peripartum cardiomyopathy (8%), anesthetic complications (2%), and amniotic fluid embolism. Nonobstetric causes include pulmonary embolism (19%), infection/sepsis (13%), stroke (5%), myocardial infarction, and trauma (4) (Table 18.1).

## Physiological Changes in Pregnancy

Physiological adaptations to pregnancy must be considered in the approach to the critically ill pregnant patient and when applying Advanced Cardiac Life Support (ACLS) guidelines. Cardiovascular

TABLE 18.1

Common Causes of Cardiac Arrest in Pregnancy

| Obstetric | Nonobstetric |
|---|---|
| Hemorrhage | Pulmonary embolism |
| Hypertensive disorders of pregnancy | Infection/sepsis |
| Idiopathic peripartum cardiomyopathy | Stroke |
| Anesthetic complications | Myocardial infarction |
| Amniotic fluid embolism | Trauma |

changes include a significant increase in cardiac output while systemic vascular resistance and arterial blood pressure are decreased compared to prepregnancy baselines. During pregnancy, the plasma volume increases by 50% with the highest rate of change at 30–34 weeks (5). This change is mediated by the increased levels of progesterone and changes in the rennin–angiotensin–aldosterone system (6). Red blood cell mass increases by up to 20%, which is relatively less than the change in plasma volume. The net result is a physiological hemodilution which decreases blood viscosity and serves as a compensatory mechanism for delivery blood loss, which averages 500–1000 $cm^3$ in a routine delivery (7).

Cardiac output (product of stroke volume and heart rate) increases by 30–50% in pregnancy (8). This is primarily due to the increase in stroke volume and, to a lesser extent, from a small increase in heart rate (9). Uterine blood flow accounts for about 2% of total cardiac output in the nonpregnant patient compared to 17% at term. This represents a blood volume of 450–750 $cm^3$/minute in the third trimester (10).

Systolic and diastolic blood pressures decrease by approximately 5–10 and 10–15 mmHg, respectively. This decrease primarily results from reduced systemic vascular resistance.

Positional changes in the pregnant patient have been shown to affect cardiac output, which is highest in the left lateral decubitus position and decreases by 25–30% while supine. This change is described as the "supine hypotensive syndrome" resulting from the compression of the inferior vena cava by the gravid uterus, which decreases venous return and reduces cardiac preload (11,12). This effect is notable after 20 weeks of gestation or when the uterine fundus is at the level of the umbilicus.

One study using magnetic resonance imaging for the assessment of maternal hemodynamics showed a 9% reduction in the left ventricular cardiac output from the supine to the left lateral position in pregnant patients after 20 weeks of gestation (3). Placing a patient in the supine position for resuscitation effectively reduces preload and cardiac output. The left lateral displacement of the uterus reduces aortocaval compression and increases cardiac output.

The elevation of the diaphragm by the gravid uterus reduces functional residual capacity (FRC), expiratory reserve volume, and residual volume in the lungs (2). Progesterone-mediated increase in minute ventilation and decreased $pCO_2$ result in a compensated physiological respiratory alkalosis. The maternal respiratory rate is unchanged; however, the maternal oxygen consumption increases. These cumulative respiratory changes predispose pregnant women to a higher risk of anoxia.

Delayed gastric emptying from the relaxation of the esophageal sphincter leads to an increased risk of aspiration during intubation. Key physiological changes in pregnancy are summarized in Table 18.2.

TABLE 18.2

Key Physiological Changes in Pregnancy

| | |
|---|---|
| Cardiac | ↑ Cardiac output (highest in left lateral decubitus position) |
| | ↑ Plasma volume |
| | ↓ Systemic vascular resistance |
| | ↓ Arterial blood pressure |
| Respiratory | ↓ FRC |
| | ↓ Expiratory reserve volume |
| | ↓ Residual volume |
| | ↑ Minute ventilation |
| Gastrointestinal | Delayed gastric emptying |

## Determining Gestational Age

A fetus is generally considered viable after 23 weeks of gestation. In a singleton gestation, the uterine fundus is palpable above the pubic symphysis after 12 weeks of gestation. At 16 weeks, it is approximately midway from the umbilicus and reaches the level of the umbilicus at 20 weeks. At 36 weeks, the fundus is at the level of the xyphoid. After 20 weeks, the gestational age is roughly estimated by the assessment of fundal height, which is the distance in centimeters from the pubic symphysis to the top of the fundus. Maternal obesity, multiple gestation, uterine fibroids, and increased amniotic fluid volume are some of the factors which can alter the reliability of estimated gestational age. Regardless of gestational age, the fetus should not be monitored during maternal resuscitation, as the maternal response, or lack of, will dictate management, not fetal condition.

## Timing of Delivery

The current consensus for delivery within 4–5 minutes of cardiac arrest in a pregnant patient is based on a landmark review published by Katz et al. (13) in 1986. The review included a series of PMCDs between 1900 and 1985. All the 42 infants delivered within the first 5 minutes of cardiac arrest had a normal neurological outcome compared to those delivered between 6 and 10, 11 and 15, and 16 and 20 minutes, respectively (13). In a follow-up series by the same authors, there were 38 cases of PMCD with 34 surviving infants. Twenty of the women had potentially treatable causes of arrest, and 13 of those were later discharged from the hospital in stable condition. There was improved maternal hemodynamic status in 12/18 women who had return of spontaneous circulation (ROSC) and blood pressure immediately after delivery (14).

The 4–5-minute rule has been challenged for its fetocentric approach, which implies the futility of maternal resuscitation. In a recent review, the authors suggest replacing the term *perimortem cesarean delivery* with *resuscitative hysterotomy* to focus on the simultaneous optimization of maternal resuscitation and improvement in fetal outcome. This paradigm shift emphasizes a "maternofetal" approach to management. It would also take into consideration the etiology of cardiac arrest and the chances of return to spontaneous circulation. Given the limitations of performing PMCD within a 4–5-minute period, they suggest that earlier consideration should be given to performing resuscitative hysterotomy to improve maternal and fetal outcomes (15). In fact, in one recent study, PMCD could not be completed within the recommended time frame despite training specific to PMCD, suggesting that the target of 4–5 minutes may not be consistently achievable. Obstacles cited included a lack of a scalpel and taking time to move the patient to the operating room (OR) (16).

Alternatively, postponing the delivery to 5 minutes should be avoided if maternal resuscitation is considered futile.

## Technique for Perimortem Cesarean Delivery

The American Heart Association published guidelines in 2015 with specific recommendations for the management of cardiac arrest in pregnancy (17). Resuscitation should be performed based on standard published guidelines. If ROSC has not occurred after 4 minutes of resuscitative efforts and manual left uterine displacement (LUD), PMCD is recommended. The preparation for possible PMCD should be initiated at the time of maternal arrest. The patient should not be moved to the OR for delivery as this decreases the quality of CPR (18). If the arrest occurs out of the hospital, transport the patient to a tertiary care center or a facility where cesarean delivery can be performed. Delays in finding surgical equipment should be avoided, and surgical consent for delivery is not required. An emergency cesarean kit is available on most labor and delivery units and should be placed at the bedside of a patient who is critically ill or with rapidly deteriorating status; however, a scalpel is the only essential tool to expedite delivery. The use of betadine or a topical antiseptic is not required but may be applied to the abdomen if available. Fetal monitoring or ultrasound is not indicated. Apply continuous manual LUD of the uterus until the fetus is delivered,

TABLE 18.3

Key Steps for PMCD

| Dos | Dont's |
|---|---|
| • Estimate gestational age by fundal height (~20 weeks at umbilicus)<br>• Proceed with PMCD after 4 minutes of resuscitation with no ROSC<br>• Perform LUD<br>• Request perimortem cesarean tray (only scalpel is required)<br>• Notify neonatology<br>• Deliver fetus and placenta<br>• Close hysterotomy or pack uterus<br>• Continue resuscitation after delivery | • Delay resuscitation to perform ultrasound to determine gestational age<br>• Monitor fetal heart tones<br>• Move patient to OR for delivery<br>• Discontinue resuscitation during delivery |

and continue chest compressions without interruption. A vertical skin incision is preferred as it allows for faster access and more exposure to the abdominal cavity. However, a Pfannenstiel incision can be performed at the surgeon's discretion. The uterus is incised using either a vertical incision or low transverse incision. The neonate is delivered and handed to the team for resuscitation (17). The placenta is delivered and the uterine incision is closed in a running layer of absorbable suture or packed if suture is not available. The abdomen should be closed in the standard fashion. Assisted vaginal delivery with forceps or vacuum is appropriate if the cervix is completely dilated and the head is at a low station. The patient's abdomen may be packed, and the patient moved to the OR after delivery at the discretion of the resuscitation team.

After delivery of the fetus, circulating blood volume and cardiac output increase as a result of autotransfusion of uteroplacental blood (19). There is improved ability to ventilate and perform effective chest compressions. After ROSC, administer broad-spectrum antibiotics for surgical prophylaxis and intravenous oxytocin to reduce postpartum bleeding. Table 18.3 and Figure 18.1 summarize key steps for performing PMCD.

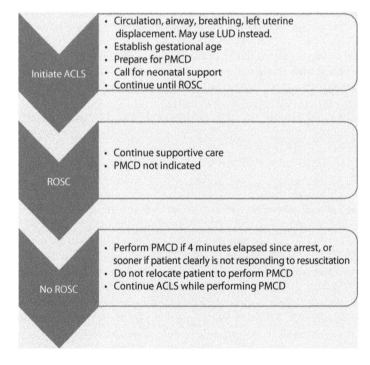

FIGURE 18.1  PMCD algorithm (ACLS, advanced cardiac life support; PMCD, perimortem cesarean delivery; ROSC, return of spontaneous circulation).

## Maternal and Fetal Outcomes

There is a direct relationship between the timing of delivery and the survival of both the mother and the neonate. A review of 38 cases of PMCD between 1998 and 2004 showed the survival of 34 infants and 13/20 mothers with reversible causes of arrest (14). A series of 53 PMCDs were reviewed to determine the mean time to delivery for maternal and fetal injury-free survival. The mean time from arrest to birth for mothers who survived cardiac arrest was 9.4 minutes compared to 24.7 minutes in the group which did not survive. Of surviving newborns, the mean time from arrest to birth was 10.1 minutes in the survivors compared to 20.3 minutes in the nonsurvivors. As expected, there was a linear relationship between injury-free survival and delivery time after arrest, for both mothers and newborns (20). PMCD leads to clear survival benefit, but the outcome is also determined by initial presenting rhythm. Asystole is associated with a worse outcome than shockable rhythms (ventricular tachycardia/ventricular fibrillation). Compliance with the 4-minute rule is variable across reported studies. In a series of 94 cases documented from 1980 to 2010, there was only 7% compliance with the 4-minute rule, but 50% neonatal survival rate even when deliveries occurred after 10 minutes (21).

PMCD is a rare event which, when performed in a timely manner, may lead to improved maternal outcome and fetal survival.

## REFERENCES

1. Mhyre JM, Tsen LC, Einav S, Kuklina EV, Leffert LR, Bateman BT. Cardiac arrest during hospitalization for delivery in the United States, 1998–2011. *J Am Soc Anesth.* 2014; 120(4):810-818.
2. Campbell TA, Sanson TG. Cardiac arrest and pregnancy. *J Emerg Trauma Shock.* 2009; 2(1):34.
3. Pritchard JA. Changes in the blood volume during pregnancy and delivery. *J Am Soc Anesth.* 1965; 26(4):393-399.
4. Carbillon L, Uzan M, Uzan S. Pregnancy, vascular tone, and maternal hemodynamics: A crucial adaptation. *Obstet Gynecol Survey.* 2000; 55(9):574-581.
5. American College of Obstetricians and Gynecologists. ACOG Practice Bulletin: Clinical management guidelines for obstetrician-gynecologists Number 76, October 2006: Postpartum hemorrhage. *Obstet Gynecol.* 2006; 108(4):1039.
6. Flo K, Wilsgaard T, Vårtun Å, Acharya G. A longitudinal study of the relationship between maternal cardiac output measured by impedance cardiography and uterine artery blood flow in the second half of pregnancy. *Obstet Anesth Digest.* 2011; 31(3):178-179.
7. Clark SL, Cotton DB, Lee W, Bishop C, Hill T, Southwick J et al. Central hemodynamic assessment of normal term pregnancy. *Am J Obstet Gynecol.* 1989; 161(6):1439-1442.
8. Gilson GJ, Samaan S, Crawford MH, Qualls CR, Curet LB. Changes in hemodynamics, ventricular remodeling, and ventricular contractility during normal pregnancy: A longitudinal study. *Obstet Gynecol.* 1997; 89(6):957-962.
9. Kinsella MS, Lohmann G. Supine hypotensive syndrome. *Obstet Gynecol.* 1994; 83(5):774-788.
10. Almeida FA, Pavan MV, Rodrigues CI. The haemodynamic, renal excretory and hormonal changes induced by resting in the left lateral position in normal pregnant women during late gestation. *BJOG: Intl J Obstet Gynaecol.* 2009; 116(13):1749-1754.
11. Rossi A, Cornette J, Johnson MR, Karamermer Y, Springeling T, Opic P et al. Quantitative cardiovascular magnetic resonance in pregnant women: Cross-sectional analysis of physiological parameters throughout pregnancy and the impact of the supine position. *J Cardiovasc Magn Reson.* 2011; 13(1):1.
12. Hegewald MJ, Crapo RO. Respiratory physiology in pregnancy. *Clin Chest Med.* 2011; 32(1):1-3.
13. Katz VL, Dotters DJ, Droegemueller W. Perimortem cesarean delivery. *Obstet Gynecol.* 1986; 68(4): 571-576.
14. Katz V, Balderston K, DeFreest M. Perimortem cesarean delivery: Were our assumptions correct? *Am J Obstet Gynecol.* 2005; 192(6):1916-1920.
15. Rose CH, Faksh A, Traynor KD, Cabrera D, Arendt KW, Brost BC. Challenging the 4-to 5-minute rule: From perimortem cesarean to resuscitative hysterotomy. *Am J Obstet Gynecol.* 2015; 213(5):653-656.

16. Jeejeebhoy FM, Zelop CM, Lipman S, Carvalho B, Joglar J, Mhyre JM et al. Cardiac arrest in pregnancy: A scientific statement from the American Heart Association. *Circulation*. 2015; 132(18):1747-1773.

17. Lipman SS, Wong JY, Arafeh J, Cohen SE, Carvalho B. Transport decreases the quality of cardiopulmonary resuscitation during simulated maternal cardiac arrest. *Anesth Analg*. 2013; 116(1):162-167.

18. Benson MD, Padovano A, Bourjeily G, Zhou Y. Perimortem cesarean delivery: Injury-free survival as a function of arrest-to-delivery interval time. *Obstet Gynecol*. 2014; 123:137S.

19. Einav S, Kaufman N, Sela HY. Maternal cardiac arrest and perimortem caesarean delivery: Evidence or expert-based? *Resuscitation*. 2012; 83(10):1191-1200.

20. Dijkman A, Huisman C, Smit M, Schutte J, Zwart J, van Roosmalen J et al. Cardiac arrest in pregnancy: Increasing use of perimortem caesarean section due to emergency skills training? *BJOG* 2010; 117:282-287.

21. Robson SC, Hunter S, Boys RJ, Dunlop W. Hemodynamic changes during twin pregnancy: A Doppler and M-mode echocardiographic study. *Am J Obstet Gynecol*. 1989; 161(5):1273-1278.

# Index

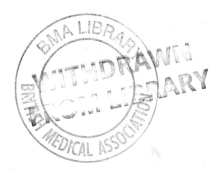